T0215318

Speech Pathology in Cultural and Linguistic Diversity

Dedication

With love and thanks to my parents for putting me on this road
and to my husband for lighting my way

Speech Pathology in Cultural and Linguistic Diversity

KIM M. ISAAC

University of Newcastle, New South Wales

W

WHURR PUBLISHERS

LONDON AND PHILADELPHIA

© 2002 Whurr Publishers Ltd
First published 2002
by Whurr Publishers Ltd
19b Compton Terrace
London N1 2UN England and
325 Chestnut Street, Philadelphia PA 19106 USA

British Library Cataloguing in Publication Data

A catalogue record for this book
is available from the British Library.

ISBN 1 86156 306 X

Reprinted 2006

Contents

Introduction

Providing speech pathology services to clients from cultural and linguistic backgrounds other than that of the majority is becoming a frequent reality in today's multicultural societies. The challenge has been issued to speech-language pathologists to provide assessment and intervention services to patients of all cultural and linguistic backgrounds in the most appropriate and effective way. How ready are we to provide services within an intercultural framework, and even more challenging, in interpreter-mediated interactions? This book aims to address the challenges faced by clinicians in intercultural and interpreter-mediated interactions by offering some ideas to assist in the development of an awareness of and sensitivity towards the complexities of intercultural interactions.

Chapter 1 discusses the basic processes of communication and the ways in which culture can influence the way we communicate verbally and non-verbally. Chapter 2 takes the process of communication further to discuss what happens when breakdown occurs, with specific reference to intercultural communication breakdown, and explores the pathway to intercultural communication competence. Chapter 3 introduces some basic issues relating to intercultural health care, including a more detailed look at the way culture influences perceptions of illness/disability and expectations of treatment. Chapter 4 extends some of the issues discussed in relation to intercultural health care, applying them to the context of speech-language pathology. This chapter takes a practical look at speech-language pathology sessions, reviewing the impact of cultural differences on assessment and treatment procedures, as well as discussing cultural attitudes towards communication disorders. Chapter 5 details some suggestions for a culturally focused speech-language pathology service, from the point of view of assessment and treatment approaches. Chapter 6 introduces the process of interpretation and includes a detailed discussion on the use of untrained interpreters. Chapter 7 presents an important factor in successful interpreter-mediated communication — the pre-session briefing. Chapter 8 reviews the potential linguistic and non-linguistic barriers to successful communication across languages. Chapter 9 presents the collaborative partnership model for working with interpreters, including a case example, and strategies for making it work. Finally, Chapter 10 explores some of the research, educational, and ethical issues related to the management of cultural and linguistic diversity for communication disorders.

The book is intended to provide an insight into intercultural communication and interpreter–clinician partnerships within the context of health care and, more specifically, speech pathology. It is more than an introduction and is suitable for clinicians who find themselves tackling the intercultural challenge everyday. The book, with its easy-to-read and practical content, is also of significant value to undergraduate students and qualified speech-language pathologists new to multicultural/multilingual contexts. The activities throughout the book reinforce the information covered in each chapter by providing an avenue for further practical consideration of the issues discussed. They can be completed individually or in groups, and are suitable for student tutorial sessions.

Chapter 1

Communication and culture

As health professionals providing a vital service to a significant proportion of children and adults living within the communities in which we work, it is inevitable that at some point in time we will find ourselves faced with the challenge of providing services to people of different cultural and linguistic backgrounds. I say *challenge* because intercultural encounters are often more complex than they are thought to be. Within the bounds of our own culture and language, interactions with others are commonly free from breakdown. This is because we share an understanding of the linguistic and cultural characteristics unique to our particular cultural group. However, interactions within our own cultural and linguistic boundaries are not *always* successful. Our attitudes, beliefs, customs, values, and interpretations of language and behaviours are shaped by the things we see, hear and learn throughout our lives. For the most part, within the same cultural group, these things will be essentially the same. However, there is room for variability and communication breakdown does occur.

Talk between friends

whenever people talk they run the risk of not being heard or understood.
(West, 1984, p. 107)

Language is complex. A single utterance can have a variety of meanings. I remember a friend's experience of reading an alternative interpretation in a sign on a Sydney train. The sign read 'When travelling at night sit near the guard's compartment marked with a blue light.' After reading this my friend burst into uncontrollable laughter, picturing a few bleary-eyed late-night travellers sitting outside the guard's compartment of the train with large blue lights on their heads. No doubt this is not the message the State Rail Authority wished to convey, and no doubt anyone reading this alternative interpretation into the sign would not believe it. What is it, then, that allows us to choose one interpretation over another? The factors that help us determine which inter-pretation of a message is the one to believe are based predominantly on our experiences and knowledge of social interaction and our context:

- knowledge about the rules of language (including content, form, and use);
- knowledge about the rules of social interaction and communication;
- knowledge about the context and environment in which the communi-cation occurs;
- knowledge or assumptions about the intent of the message.

In the above example of the sign in the train, it can easily be assumed that my friend's alternative interpretation is not the correct one. Although the structure of the message allows both interpretations, our knowledge of the context (train travel), assumed intention of the message (to promote safety), and rules for social interaction (that walking around with a blue light on your head may be seen as inappropriate) all contribute to the decision that this interpretation is nothing more than a parody. Let us consider a different example.

> *If a child is a late talker it is always worthwhile ruling out hearing as one of the problems.*

As speech-language pathologists (SLPs), we know that this statement means that children who are late to develop speech or language may have an under-lying hearing impairment, and therefore a hearing assessment is advisable. Thus, we know that delayed language development can be contributed to by hearing impairment. But, how do we know which one is the problem and which is the contributing factor? As SLPs, our experience and education tells us. What now if we look at another sentence:

> *If a child is a spiddish woot it is always worthwhile ruling out dobblehob as one of the problems.*

What does this mean? Does *spiddish woot* contribute to *dobblehob* or does it occur because of *dobblehob*? You may take the same structure as the previous sentence to be true, that is, that *spiddish woot* is contributed to by *dobblehob*. However, if I tell you that *spiddish woot* means *sweet tooth* and *dobblehob* means *cavities* then the sentence would read:

> *If a child is a sweet tooth it is always worthwhile ruling out cavities as one of the problems.*

The structure of the sentence remains the same, but we have to choose a different interpretation: that *dobblehob* can be contributed to by *spiddish woot.* We have to do this because our knowledge of dental hygiene tells us that sugar can contribute to the development of caries. So, the interpretation we choose depends on our understanding of the content and our knowledge of how those key words relate to each other.

Food for thought

How often have you experienced a breakdown in communication with someone you know well? Reflect back on a time when a miscommunication occurred — what was the cause of the problem? *If you are unable to identify a particular episode of communication breakdown, listen for an example in the conversations between other people, or in your own interactions.*

Activity 1.1

Consider the following examples of communication breakdown. What is causing each misunderstanding?

> 1. A: Do you have the time?
> (gloss: Tell me the time)
> B: Yes.

In this example, Speaker A is asking Speaker B for the time. However, the request is phrased using an indirect (and perhaps more polite) form, which has been interpreted literally by Speaker B. Some cultures use indirect request forms to indicate politeness, whereas other cultures do not use such indirect forms and are therefore at risk of interpreting such a request literally. Similarly, use of a direct request may be at risk of being interpreted as impolite in a culture where politeness forms are commonly used and expected.

> 2. A (to a fellow passenger on a long-distance coach [bus]): Ask the driver what time we get to Birmingham.
> B (to driver): Could you tell me when we get to Birmingham, please?
> Driver: Don't worry, love, it's a big place - I don't think it's possible to miss it!
> (Thomas, 1983, p.296)

In this example, the communication breakdown has occurred because of the double meaning and ambiguity surrounding the word 'when'. Both Speaker B and the driver understand that the request is for the arrival time, however the immediacy of the need is ambiguous. Speaker B requests the time, expecting an immediate response - a prediction of what time the bus is due to arrive in Birmingham. The driver, on the other hand, interprets the request as a need to know when the bus arrives in Birmingham at the time of arrival, perhaps assuming that the woman is fearful of missing her stop. This difference in interpretation may be due, in part, to individual experiences. For example, the driver may be more familiar with passengers asking him to tell them when the bus has arrived at a particular stop, as opposed to a predicted time of arrival.

Culture and communication

The way in which a message is expressed by one or understood by another is influenced by a range of factors:

- sociodemographic factors (for example, age, gender, level of education, area of residence/upbringing, social status);
- past experiences (for example, upbringing, education, jobs, social interactions);
- knowledge of pragmatics (for example, how to behave/communicate in a given situation and how the behaviours/communication of others should be understood);
- the content, including intended effect, of the message spoken or heard;
- the context within which the communication/interaction takes place.

All these factors will be influenced and defined by culture (see Figure 1.1). Interactions within the bounds of our own language and culture will be less influenced by cultural variability, but even those small differences in what we see, hear, and learn can alter the way in which we interpret the language and behaviours of others.

What if we are interacting with someone from a different culture? Let's consider two popular models of communication that have been described in the literature – the code model and the inferential model.

The code model describes the historical theory of communication, which suggests that messages are encoded into a signal, which can then be decoded by the receiver. Sperber and Wilson (1995) review the code model for human verbal communication and describe it as thoughts that are linguistically encoded into mutually intelligible acoustic signals (for example, speech), which are then transmitted through the air, possibly distorted by noise, before being received and linguistically decoded into a matching thought. Just as the colour of a traffic light is unambiguously encoded and decoded into a thought which informs us to stop or go, the code model for verbal communication implies an unambiguous understanding of the signals being transmitted. But, can communication be explained so simplistically, or is it a more complex phenomenon?

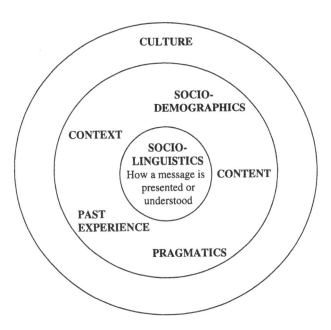

Figure 1.1. Cultural and linguistic influences on communication.

Figure 1.1 hypothesizes that the way in which a message is presented or understood depends on a myriad of social, cultural, and linguistic factors. This hypothesis is also discussed by Sperber and Wilson. A new model for communication was being proposed in the literature. Sperber and Wilson reviewed this new development in their discussion and termed it the inferential model of communication. It suggests that communication consists of the interpretation of inference, so that the speaker's message, when linguistically encoded, is decoded by the hearer according to their standards of 'truthfulness, informativeness, comprehensibility, and so on' (p. 13). Thus, the inferential model accounts for communication between people of different language or cultural background, who may have different assumptions and standards with which to interpret the meaning of an utterance. This inferential model of communication may be represented as in Figure 1.2.

Taking the simplest form of interaction, the dyad, it can be seen that both partners have their own assumptions, including standards, of communication based on their social, cultural, and linguistic makeup (labelled A1 and A2). The assumptions of each partner are not exactly the same, thus they are offset, with a common overlapping area representing those that are the same. A message will be successfully transmitted if the assumptions with which the message was presented match the assumptions with which the message was

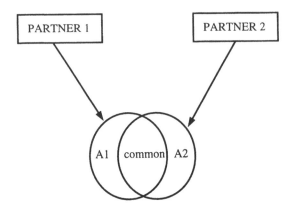

Figure 1.2. The inferential model of communication as described by Sperber and Wilson (1995).

understood, thereby drawing from the 'common' area. However, since the assumptions of each partner are not identical, it is inevitable that communication breakdown can occur (Sperber and Wilson, 1995). While flying to America recently I experienced an unresolved communication breakdown with one of the flight attendants. Not long after the plane left Sydney a flight attendant came around offering drinks. I asked for a lemonade (for me this meant a clear, carbonated, lemon-flavoured drink). However, I was politely told that she didn't have any. I was somewhat bewildered by that, but instead had a Coke. Later she returned to offer another drink — I thought, 'well, if they don't have any lemonade, surely they'll have a lemon squash' (for me this meant a carbonated lemon-flavoured drink, which is usually lemon in colour). The flight attendant looked at me with a puzzled face and repeated that they didn't have any. Even more bewildered now, I ordered another Coke. It wasn't until I arrived in America that my friend explained that lemonade means freshly squeezed lemon juice (usually diluted and sweetened). Lemon squash is not a term generally used in North America, and perhaps the flight attendant interpreted this literally as *squashed lemon* (and, therefore, lemon juice). Lemon juice is definitely not what I was wanting — I should have asked for a Sprite or 7-Up. So, despite our relatively similar cultures and same language background, the flight attendant and I had an unresolved communication breakdown, with the meanings of 'lemonade' and 'lemon squash' not being part of those assumptions and standards we share. On the surface it may appear that this is a breakdown due to lack of shared word meaning. A deeper analysis suggests a cultural component. The way in which words are used to express meaning is culturally defined. When asking for a *lemonade* or *lemon squash* I was referring to the generic category of lemon-flavoured carbonated drinks. However, the flight attendant perhaps expected drinks to be labelled by brand name (such as 7-Up, Sprite) and therefore interpreted my request according to her own specific knowledge of the term *lemonade*.

This is where the challenge in achieving effective intercultural communication lies. What do we know about other cultures? Unless we have had a significant experience with a particular culture, most of our knowledge probably comes from what we see and hear, such as eating habits, dress, customs, and rituals. That is, behaviours that are externalized. Battle (1993) describes these as explicit cultural characteristics. She also identifies implicit cultural characteristics, those that are internalized within the individual and/or culture. These would include family and social roles, religious beliefs and practices, child rearing practices, attitudes towards health and illness, attitudes towards education, perception of and reaction to authority, use and interpretation of non-verbal behaviours (for example, eye contact, personal space), and learning styles.

Cultural iceberg

An interesting analogy, described by Goodman (1994), is to think of culture as an iceberg (see Figure 1.3). The part of the iceberg seen above the water represents the explicit cultural characteristics. Under the water is the mass of the ice that cannot be seen, representing the implicit cultural characteristics. It is this mass of ice that is the most threatening to the success of a ship's voyage. Similarly, being oblivious to the presence of implicit cultural characteristics can be dangerous practice in any intercultural interaction. Thus, to communicate and interact effectively interculturally we must know something about the culture of our communication partner, particularly the implicit characteristics.

Irwin (1996, p. 134) states that 'The ability to negotiate culture and communicate effectively and comfortably interculturally depends upon culture learning.' But, how do we 'culture learn'? We can 'culture learn' by:

- understanding the characteristics and behaviours of others;
- not just mimicking the behaviours of others;
- being aware of our own cultural idiosyncrasies.

Thus, we need to develop an understanding of and sensitivity towards the behaviours of people from cultures other than our own, as opposed to mimicking those behaviours without an understanding of the meanings or implications involved. It is suggested that we try to understand ourselves before we try to understand others, and in that way we'll be more able to understand the differences. It does not mean that all aspects and all

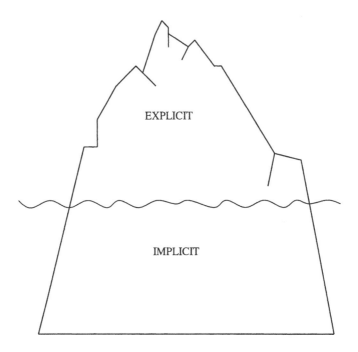

Figure 1.3. The cultural iceberg as described by Goodman (1994) showing implicit and explicit cultural characteristics.

behaviours of a culture be learned. In contrast, it advocates a general awareness of cultural differences, where to find out more information, and how to negotiate or discuss differences in culturally sensitive ways (Irwin, 1996).

Cultural influences on communication

Culture can be influenced by many things. It can be influenced by where we live or the community group with which we identify. It can be influenced by our upbringing, our experiences and opportunities, schooling, peer relationships, and social norms and expectations. It can be influenced by the media, including television, radio, books, magazines, newspapers and movies. It can be influenced by religion and family roles and values. These are just some examples of social and experiential factors that can influence the development of our cultural identity.

Similarly, culture can influence our ways of being — the ways we communicate, interact, and behave. Culture can influence our concept of individualism or collectivism, social equality, food, eating habits and dress style. It can influence our communication style and social behaviour and the way in which we modify these to suit different contexts — settings and communication partners. It influences the way we treat other people, our concept of gender roles, our sense of competitiveness and assertiveness, and self-confidence. Culture influences our non-verbal behaviours, our attitudes towards health and illness/disability, our attitudes towards education and work, as well as our child-rearing practices and family roles and values. Culture is dynamic and vast. It is everywhere and cannot be avoided. Although you may think of culture as something belonging to other groups of people, it also belongs to you. Everyone has a culture and everyone is influenced by culture.

Food for thought

Can you identify what your culture is? What are your beliefs, attitudes and values? How has your culture influenced your life and way of being? Can you identify any differences with your friends/colleagues? What do you think has influenced those differences?

Non-verbal communication

As already discussed, culture influences many aspects of our ways of being, including behaviour and communication styles. Non-verbal communication accounts for a significant proportion of any communicative interaction. It includes eye contact, smiling, laughing, how we sit, where we sit, physical proximity and physical touching, hand gestures, facial expression and body language. It is part of every communicative act we perform and conveys specific meaning that may confirm or contradict our verbal message. But, just as verbal communication is influenced by culture, so too is non-verbal communication. There is the potential for discrepancy across cultures in the way a non-verbal signal is used and in the way it is understood by the receiver, giving rise to several potential barriers to the success of an intercultural interaction:

* we may inadvertently send the wrong message;
* we risk causing offence or embarrassment; and
* we may miss subtle non-verbal cues that may indicate the speaker's true intent.

We cannot assume that non-verbal behaviours will be understood as we intend by people from culturally diverse backgrounds. Similarly, we cannot attribute meaning to the non-verbal behaviours of others using our own culturally defined understanding. Consider the following examples:

American teachers of Asian students often misinterpret silence on the part of their students. Asian students may not speak out in class as much as their American counterparts. American teachers are used to students who willingly answer questions and speak up in front of others. Therefore, the American teachers may interpret the silence of the Asian students as a lack of interest or dullness when, in fact, their silence is really a result of respect for the teacher and a reluctance to stand apart from their classmates.

(Singelis, 1994, p. 280)

Richard Nixon fell into this pitfall when visiting Latin America. On arriving, Nixon gave the A-Okay sign. However, this gesture has a very different meaning in Latin America. Putting the thumb and forefinger together in a circle and extending the other fingers is an obscene gesture (indicating the female genitalia) in Latin America. Richard Nixon was very embarrassed and the Latin Americans were very offended.

(Singelis, 1994, p. 280)

Eye contact is an unavoidable non-verbal signal — even closing your eyes in an attempt to avoid eye contact during an interaction conveys meaning — but eye contact can have significantly different meanings attributed to it. For example, prolonged eye contact, made with individuals who are relative strangers, can be understood as an indication of anger and hostility, rudeness, disrespect (especially if the stranger is an elder), or it can be viewed as a sign of interest. Smiling can indicate happiness, embarrassment, apology, or can hide feelings of pain or discomfort. A raised thumb is used to indicate approval in Ireland, yet the same gesture reflects an insult in Greece (MacLachlan, 1997). Silence is another non-verbal behaviour that can convey different meanings across cultures. In many Anglo-European cultures (for example, in North America, Britain, Australia and some parts of Europe) silence in response to another's conversational turn is likely to be interpreted as misunderstanding. This interpretation is usually made within a few seconds after which the speaker may attempt to repair the breakdown — 'Do you understand?' 'Maybe that wasn't clear enough . . .', 'What I mean is . . .' and so on. In contrast, a listener from Japan or an indigenous Australian, for example, places greater value on silence, and uses it to convey respect for what the speaker has said. It is often a sign of thought and shows that the listener is preparing a suitable response. Many Anglo-Europeans may find these silences uncomfortable. They may try to jump in to repair the perceived breakdown, to the frustration of the listener.

Studies show variation in the extent to which non-verbal behaviour accounts for total communication. However, there is consensus among researchers that non-verbal communication is more powerful than its verbal counterpart, with estimates reported in the literature varying from 65% to

93% of total communication (Singelis, 1994). The reasons why non-verbal communication may be more effective and powerful than verbal communication have been described by Singelis. He suggests that the multichannelled nature of non-verbal communication has a more powerful impact because the non-verbal message can be conveyed by visual, auditory, olfactory, and tactile channels. Often a non-verbal message is conveyed by a combination of channels. For example, facial expression, tone of voice, and body posture will, together, convey a much stronger message than the verbal output (words) alone. In every culture and country around the world non-verbal communication is observed to develop before verbal communication. Babies are able to successfully indicate their basic needs and wants by using variations in vocalizations and gestures, long before they learn to use words. Finally, Singelis suggests that non-verbal communication is unmediated — that is, it is a more direct form of communication, not necessarily requiring any encoding or decoding processes, and so may be seen as more reliable or trustworthy compared with verbal communication.

However, as the examples above demonstrate, non-verbal behaviours are not always common across cultural groups. In addition, people are often able to control the way in which they express feelings non-verbally based on their culture-bound rules of what is appropriate in a given context. For example, it may be appropriate to laugh in private amongst close friends and family, but inappropriate in public. In intercultural contexts, it can be dangerous to continue assuming non-verbal behaviours are a reliable insight into someone's true feelings, given that non-verbal behaviours can be regulated to suit different contexts and that meanings can vary (sometimes considerably) across cultures. Thus, in intercultural contexts it may be necessary to go through encoding and decoding processes, in order to actively examine the meaning behind unexpected non-verbal behaviours. Applying our own culturally determined rules in intercultural contexts may result in false negative judgements about the person who has used the unexpected non-verbal behaviour. Consider the following example,

A: Have you experienced this pain for long?
B (looking down at the floor): No.

In this example, A may assume that B is intentionally avoiding eye contact and may interpret this as an attempt to hide the truth, when in fact B may be avoiding direct eye contact with A as a sign of respect for his/her authority. If A applies his/her own culturally determined rule for avoiding eye contact, he or she may assume that B is hiding something. In response, A may pursue a line of questioning aimed at revealing the 'truth' — an inappropriate response if B has already answered honestly.

Summary

This chapter has explored the dynamic relationship between culture and communication. Numerous examples from the literature and personal experience illustrated the way in which culture can influence the success of a communicative interaction. As communicators, the way in which we express ourselves or understand others is determined by our past experiences and knowledge about social-cultural rules for appropriate behaviour and communicative interaction in given contexts. Yet, our experiences (and how we interpret them), pragmatic knowledge, communicative content, and (to a lesser extent) communicative context are culturally defined. Similarly, rules for communication and interaction based on gender, age, and educational or societal status are also influenced by culture. An inferential model of communication was discussed to clarify the very personal nature of communication within culture. This model proposed that every individual develops assumptions, standards, and beliefs about the world (including rules for communication and behaviour) which are based on their unique life experiences. Thus, there can be considerable cultural variation between people, even when culture and language are superficially the same. When cultural experiences are obviously different, successful communicative exchange becomes more problematic, with greater opportunity for breakdown. Non-verbal aspects of communication and implicit cultural characteristics are additional factors contributing to the complexity of intercultural communication.

In intercultural exchanges, it is important to realize that cultural competence does not necessarily come from a thorough understanding of the cultural and communicative features of any, or all, community groups. Indeed, given the intricate nature of culture, including considerable in-group variation, full understanding would be a rare achievement, unless you are an accepted member of the ethnic group in question. Rather, a developed *awareness* of cultural difference and its potential to effect communicative behaviour is paramount. Awareness of your own beliefs, values, and perceptions as well as insight into how culture has influenced your personal and professional style is another key element in facilitating cultural sensitivity. You'll remember it was suggested that we try to understand ourselves before we try to understand others, so that we have a heightened awareness and appreciation of our differences. Finally, it is essential to consider the reality of in-group variation. Assuming that all members of a specific cultural group will behave in the same way or have the same beliefs, values, and perceptions may only result in false stereotyping of group members. Contact with members of other cultural groups, personal experiences (including educational, professional, and social), and levels of acculturation or assimilation have the potential to vary considerably across the group. Our awareness of cultural difference needs to be aimed at the individual level rather than the group level. Thus, exploring cultural difference through assessment procedures is an important consideration in clinical practice. This will be explored in detail in later chapters.

CHAPTER 2

Miscommunication

So far we have looked at verbal and non-verbal communication across cultures and we have touched on the potential difficulties that can arise in intercultural interactions. These difficulties or breakdowns in communication can be termed *miscommunications*. Traditionally, miscommunication was thought to be due to the use of false, misleading, or vague information. This can certainly be the case — an ambiguous or incorrect message will have a greater chance of resulting in communication breakdown than a true and well-formed message. However, even true and well-formed messages can result in misunderstanding. So then, what causes this type of miscommunication?

The inferential model of communication (Figure 1.2) shows how our culture (experiences, attitudes, beliefs, and so forth) influences the development of unique standards and assumptions about what we expect from and understand of our world. Thus, the way we present a message and the way we understand a message from someone else will depend on our culture, expectations and standards. Even using the same language does not guarantee successful communication because culture influences so many aspects of our life. Consider this next example:

> If an American were to come home from work and say that during the day she gave a speech and it 'bombed' and afterwards the proposal she had been working on for 6 months was 'tabled' at the executive board meeting, it would be clear to most Americans that this executive had had a pretty miserable day. To the British, however, she had a marvelous day. In the United States, to have your speech bomb is synonymous with disaster, it was a horrible failure, whereas in Britain it was a splendid success. In the United States, to have your motion tabled implies that it has been put *off* the table with no further discussion at that time, whereas in Britain having your motion tabled means it is being put *on* the table for discussion.
>
> (Goodman, 1994, p. 44)

In Australia there would be yet another interpretation of this woman's day — a good and bad day. Her speech was a disaster but her motion was put on the table for discussion at the board meeting. Thus, even between these relatively similar cultures, which all share the same language, there is potential for miscommunication to occur.

Food for thought

How many additional words, phrases, or behaviours can you identify that have different meanings across cultures?

Motivation, knowledge, and skill

It has been proposed that there are three components of communication, which influence the way we communicate/interact and the way we attribute meaning to the communicative attempts of other people. Spitzberg (1991) suggests that the three components — motivation, knowledge and skill — are seen as 'additive individual competencies' (p. 22). That is, a combined increase in motivation, knowledge and skill has the effect of increasing perceived communication competence and conversational satisfaction.

In any communicative interaction, the degree to which the interaction is successful or effective depends on these three components of communication. As a communicative partner participating in a communicative exchange I need to be motivated to communicate clearly, effectively, and appropriately; I need to know how to communicate clearly, effectively, and appropriately; and I need to have the skill to use those behaviours which will make my communicative turns clear, effective, and appropriate. If I am faced with participating in a communicative exchange I feel uncomfortable and/or anxious about, my motivation or my desire to participate in that exchange would be reduced. I may feel anxious or uncomfortable because of reduced knowledge or skill about how to best participate in that exchange. For example, as a predominantly paediatric therapist I have had very little to do with the assessment or treatment of adult laryngectomies. I do not pretend to have the level of knowledge or skill required to assess or treat a patient effectively. I would feel anxious and uncomfortable in providing a service to this patient, knowing my level of knowledge and skill, and thus I would be less motivated to be involved in the assessment or treatment interaction. I may in fact seek to refer the patient on to someone who has the knowledge and skill to provide the patient with the most appropriate and effective service. However, if I am unable to refer the patient on, I would ensure that I attempt to develop my knowledge and skill in the area of laryngectomy care by consulting with other professionals and researching into assessment and treatment approaches prior to seeing the patient. Having this improved knowledge base will help me to feel more comfortable with my skills and therefore less anxious and more motivated to participate in the session. Thus, in the same way, I can improve my level of communication competence by adjusting my level of motivation, knowledge and skill.

Influence on intercultural communication competence

The three components of communication can also be applied to intercultural encounters. If you have had limited experience communicating across cultures you might feel anxious and uncertain about participating in such an intercultural exchange. You might feel that you lack the knowledge and skill required to communicate effectively and appropriately interculturally and may, therefore, have less of a desire to enter into the communicative interaction. The weaker we perceive our knowledge and skill to be, the more anxious and uncertain we are likely to feel about the interaction, and the less motivated we will be to participate in it. If we enter into a communicative exchange at this point, it is likely to be ineffective and inappropriate. Thus, we need to improve our communication competence so that we feel less anxious about communicating interculturally.

Gudykunst (1993) suggests that the development of intercultural communication competence is influenced by motivational factors (such as our openness to new information) and knowledge factors (such as awareness of alternative meanings). He describes how people can be categorized into one of two groups for each of these components of communication, based on their openness to unfamiliar behaviours and their awareness of potential alternatives in meaning. He identifies the two categories as:

- certainty versus uncertainty orientation, and
- broad versus narrow categorization.

Certainty versus uncertainty orientation

People who are categorized as *certainty oriented* are comfortable with what is familiar — comfortable with what they are certain about. They do not tend to search for different meanings to attribute to observed behaviours, being satisfied with their old, familiar beliefs. They are less able to evaluate themselves, their behaviours, and their expectations of others. People who are categorized as *uncertainty oriented*, on the other hand, are comfortable with what is unfamiliar — comfortable with what they are uncertain about. These people are more aware that an observed behaviour may have another meaning. They are able to evaluate themselves, their behaviours, and their expectations of others in an open and constructive way. Gudykunst (1993) suggests that certainty-oriented people are more anxious and uncertain about interacting with strangers, whereas uncertainty-oriented people are able to reduce their levels of anxiety and uncertainty because they are more aware of potential differences and why they exist. In intercultural interactions, people who have taken the time to develop a sensitivity to other ways of communicating and behaving, recognizing that their way is only one out of many, are more likely to have a successful and mutually fulfilling communicative interaction.

Broad versus narrow categorization

An awareness and understanding of what needs to be done to communicate competently, what Spitzberg (1991) termed *knowledge*, is also an important factor in competent intercultural interactions. Gudykunst reviews how people can be divided into two distinct groups according to the way in which they judge the behaviours of another. People who are *broad categorizers* understand that they cannot use their own cultural values to judge the behaviour of another, understanding that there can be a variety of ways to interpret such behaviours. These people are broad-minded with an open awareness of alternate interpretations. In contrast, people who are *narrow categorizers* tend to be less aware of the existence of different interpretations and are, therefore, likely to judge another's behaviour based on their own cultural values and standards of what is appropriate in given contexts. These people are narrow minded, with closed views about what is right and appropriate. Narrow categorizing can result in *false negative* judgements. That is, assigning a negative judgement based on your own standards of what is appropriate behaviour, when in fact the behaviour is appropriate in the other person's culture. Consider the following example:

A: Is it a good restaurant?
B: Of course.

(Thomas, 1983, p. 305)

If the above example is assumed to occur between two people of English-speaking cultural background, then speaker A could take offence at speaker B's seemingly abrupt response, interpreting the 'of course' to mean 'what a stupid question — of course it's a good restaurant!' If, however, the interaction takes place between two people of Russian-speaking cultural background, then they would understand that speaker B's response means nothing more than 'yes, it is a good restaurant' (Thomas, 1983). In an interaction where speaker A is of English-speaking cultural background and speaker B of Russian-speaking cultural background, two scenarios can arise. If speaker A is a *narrow categorizer* and interprets speaker B's response in the light of his/her own cultural values, then he/she may very well take offence at B's seemingly abrupt style, where no offence was intended — a

false negative judgement. As a broad categorizer, speaker A may understand that there can be a variety of ways in which B's response can be interpreted, and may wait for some other sign that could clarify B's attitude.
Consider this next example:

A: Hi. How are you? I haven't seen you for months.
B: Yeah. I've been working overseas.
A: Oh, I see. (Smiling) Gee, you look so fat!
B: Oh . . . I . . . um . . .
A: Look at your cheeks — (laughing) so fat!
B: (puzzled and irritated) Well, yes, I suppose I . . .

(O'Sullivan, 1994, pp. 104–5)

What is happening in this example? If I was to interpret this according to what I believe are Australian standards, then I may well believe that speaker A is rude and tactless in making comments about speaker A's weight gain. In doing this, though, I am acting as a narrow categorizer, and by not understanding the intention of speaker A, I may be assigning them a false negative judgement. In fact, speaker A has a cultural background in which weight gain is synonymous with good health, and therefore intends to compliment speaker B. In this example, both speakers are narrow categorizers because they are unaware of the potential for alternate meanings for weight gain, instead using their own culturally defined understanding. Speaker B seems somewhat offended at A's comments and has probably assigned a false negative judgement. Speaker A can also be classified as certainty oriented because he or she does not seem able to evaluate the comments about weight gain according to B's reaction. The solution to this interaction would be to avoid quick assumptions based on your own cultural values, beliefs, and standards, and try to see where the other person is coming from, questioning their meaning to repair the breakdown, if unsure.

In intercultural speech-language pathology interactions we want to strive towards being uncertainty oriented and broad categorizing by having an awareness of alternative interpretations of communicative and social behaviours. We can do this by developing an understanding of the culture of the patient (the term *patient* will be used throughout the text to refer to people who seek health care and/or speech-language pathology services, regardless of the setting this service is provided in); our own stereotypes, prejudices, values, assumptions, and beliefs; and our perceptions of the differences and similarities between the two cultural groups.

However, as many cultural characteristics are implicit it can be difficult to develop an understanding or awareness of other cultures and how communicative and social behaviours should be interpreted. Thus, there is the danger of applying false negative judgements about the behaviour of our communicative partner. To avoid situations such as this, it can be useful to speak with someone who has a deep understanding of the other culture (such as an interpreter, community leader for that particular cultural group, a bicultural colleague or friend), or by reading relevant literature that details some of the explicit and implicit cultural characteristics (for example, Battle, 1993; Bebout and Arthur, 1992; Cheng, 1989a; Irwin, 1996; Lynch and Hanson, 1998; Matsuda, 1989; Meyers, 1992; O'Sullivan, 1994; Patston, 1991; Singelis, 1994; Stevens and Fletcher, 1989).

No one could ever have a thorough understanding of every characteristic of every culture on earth, but to increase our chances of succeeding interculturally we need to have:

- an awareness of the potential for differences to exist;
- an open mind so we can analyse and appraise, rather than critique; and
- knowledge of where to access information.

The pages at the end of this book can be used to keep a record of resources and contacts you have found useful in obtaining such cultural information.

Developing intercultural communication competence

When motivation, knowledge, and skill exist their combined force is believed to have the effect of minimizing feelings of anxiety and uncertainty about the communicative interaction being entered into (Gudykunst, 1993). In intercultural interactions, however, motivation, knowledge, and skill are at greater risk of not being sufficiently developed. The private nature of implicit cultural characteristics, our own stereotypes and prejudices, our degree of acceptance of unfamiliar behaviours and interpretations of those behaviours, our degree of flexibility in the interaction style we assume, and our motivations for entering into an intercultural interaction will all influence the degree to which we achieve intercultural communication competence. If we have little knowledge and skill we are likely to have greater anxiety and uncertainty about the interaction. High levels of anxiety and uncertainty are likely to make it harder to assume a flexible position in terms of inter-action/communication style and may cloud our ability to perceive other interpretations for behaviour. Thus, high anxiety and uncertainty can make us poor communicators in intercultural encounters. Negative experiences in intercultural encounters may only serve to reinforce our low levels of motivation, knowledge and skill, causing rising anxiety and uncertainty and a downward spiral in communication competence.

How can that downward spiral be broken then? Generally, we need a developed awareness of our own culture and the cultural influences on our communication and behaviour. We need to examine our motivations and our flexibility in accepting alternate interpretations to behaviour. We could also examine our knowledge, or lack of knowledge, about the other's culture and cultural influences on communication and behaviour. Finally, we should be aware of our skills in being able to interact/communicate competently interculturally.

More specifically, we need to develop our flexibility for accepting alternative interpretations (becoming broad categorizers and uncertainty oriented). We need to raise our knowledge of other cultures through reading, researching, sharing experiences with colleagues, and speaking with people who know — that is, we need to culture learn. We also need to raise our skill level in the ability to communicate/interact with people from cultures other than our own.

CHAPTER 3

Intercultural health care

Health care encounters can be fraught with difficulty and communication breakdown even when the clinician and patient share the same cultural and language background. Shuy (1976, p. 376) reported on some medical miscommunications involving doctors and patients of the same cultural and language background.

> Physician: Have you ever had a history of cardiac arrest in your family?
> Patient: We never had no trouble with the police.
>
> Physician: How about varicose veins?
> Patient: Well, I have veins, but I don't know if they're close or not.

So, why has this miscommunication occurred? You will recall the inferential model of communication (Sperber and Wilson, 1995), which suggests that each individual has unique views, values, and standards influenced by their own life experiences. In the two examples above, the patient and doctor share the same broad culture and language, but do not share the knowledge associated with the culture of medicine. The doctor uses discipline-specific terminology (cardiac arrest, varicose veins) which the patient does not understand. In response, the patient interprets the doctor's words using their existing knowledge base — focusing on 'arrest' for 'cardiac arrest' and hearing 'varicose' as 'very close'. However, mishearings and misunderstandings of jargon terms do not solely account for miscommunication in health-care contexts. Indeed, factors relating to the socially defined roles and expectations of health-care encounters can also influence the way in which clinicians and patients communicate, which in turn influence the success of the health-care encounter, as measured by satisfaction, outcomes and, perhaps, patient compliance. Health-care encounters are generally *unequal* encounters, with the health professional possessing specialist knowledge and skill. This tends to place them in a more powerful role since they are able to determine how the health-care service will be provided (Pauwels, 1995). In any health-care encounter it is generally expected that the health professional will be able to determine the patient's problem and provide appropriate treatment strategies. Expectations of how this is done, though, will vary greatly across cultural groups. Pauwels suggests that in a biomedical context the health professional is usually expected to:

• ask questions about the patient's presenting condition;
• provide information about procedures and examinations;
• provide information about the patient's problem, causes and treatment options;
• provide advice or counselling, as required.

The patient, in this same health-care context, is usually expected to:

• present the problem or complaint to the health professional;
• answer questions about the problem or complaint;
• ask questions about the problem, procedures, or treatment techniques;
• provide feedback regarding the effect of procedures and treatment.

Within same-language/same-culture interactions, uneven power distribution and mismatched expectations can result in communication breakdown, dissatisfaction, and possibly misdiagnosis. Pauwels presents five common complaints associated with doctor–patient communication, which can also be applied to communication between patients and other health professionals. She suggests that patients often feel that health professionals do not have the time to answer questions or discuss their concerns; that health professionals do not really listen; that health professionals do not offer adequate explanation for the patient's problem; that health professionals use technical language which patients do not understand; and that health professionals do not respect patients' individual knowledge, beliefs, and differences.

When the health professional and patient do not share a common cultural background, the risk of communication breakdown, feelings of dissatisfaction, non-compliance, poor outcomes, and potential misdiagnosis must increase. Cultural diversity in health-care encounters can result in mismatched expectations and perceptions about:

• health professional and patient roles;
• assessment/examination procedures; and
• the cause of the problem and appropriate treatment approaches.

Food for thought

When communicating with patients from cultures other than your own, what aspects of the biomedical approach to health-care encounters may result in breakdown?

In answering this question, we need to consider how cultural beliefs may influence perception of illness/disability and expectations about health-care services. We have described a typical biomedical health-care encounter as an unequal power distribution with the health professional holding the majority of power over the course and content of health-care procedures and over the control of the communication routines which occur as part of the encounter. That is, health professionals generally maintain a higher degree of control over what is said and contribute more to the communicative exchange than do patients. Despite this imbalance, health professionals using a biomedical approach will generally encourage patients to become active in decision-making and goal setting for their own health care. However, cultural beliefs may mean that health professionals are revered by some patients and are thought to possess almost mystical powers. It may be considered unnecessary to describe symptoms to health professionals because their skill and knowledge should allow them to diagnose the patient with minimal examination. Similarly, it may be considered inappropriate for the patient to question, or even participate in, the discussion about examination or treatment options, even if the patient disagrees with the options. Questions of a personal nature, especially if asked too early in the interview, and physical examinations may be considered inappropriate or even offensive, particularly when the patient and health professional are of different genders. Gender differences may also impact on the perceived status of the health professional. Female health professionals may be given less respect and trust by male patients, especially if the patient is older.

Perceptions of illness/disability

Culture influences our perceptions about health, illness, and disability, and particularly our perceptions of what causes illness or disability and our expectations about assessment and intervention. Working in the health field, we frequently come into contact with people who suffer from illness or disability to varying degrees. It may be a disability of communication only, or there may be a physical, emotional, or social impairment as the primary disability, as an associated factor, or as an unrelated problem. Whatever the case, differences in perception of what has caused the illness or disability may result in potential barriers to the assessment and/or treatment approach.

Working from a biomedical model, illness or disability is usually attributed to factors that are believed to have a scientific basis. For example:

- exposure to allergens (for example, pollens, foods, animal fur);
- viral or bacterial infection;
- genetic inheritance;
- substance abuse;
- compromised immune system;
- another health problem;
- traumatic injury;
- life stresses;
- changes in environment and diet.

A more traditional model may attribute illness or disability to factors based on religious, philosophical or cultural beliefs. For example:

- angry ancestors or spirits;
- broken traditions;
- punishment for sins committed in this life, a previous life, or by ancestors;
- broken taboos;
- improper diet;
- unreleased and excessive emotion;
- laziness;
- imbalance of inner forces (for example, yin and yang).

Chan provides some examples of traditional perceptions of the causes of illness and disability:

> One mother, a recent Chinese immigrant and parent of a child with Down Syndrome, attributed her daughter's hypotonia to her failure to drink adequate amounts of beef bone soup during pregnancy.

> One mother, for example (who was ethnic Chinese-Vietnamese), worked throughout her pregnancy as a seamstress and thus frequently used scissors; she felt this caused her daughter's unique hand anomaly, characterised by fused fingers and a split thumb. This attribution is consistent with the traditional belief that women should avoid using scissors, knives, and other sharp objects during pregnancy for fear of causing a miscarriage or birth defects such as a cleft lip . . .

> Another mother (Chinese from Hong Kong) of a child with a cleft palate and other congenital facial anomalies assumed that these were due to her having seen horror films and pictures of evil gods during the initial stages of her pregnancy.

> A Cambodian father attributed his daughter's 'club' foot to an incident when he and his wife were escaping as refugees through the jungles of Thailand; in an attempt to hunt and kill a bird with a rock, he instead only wounded its claw and leg.

> (Chan, 1992, pp. 225-9)

Delbar (1999) described a case of an Ethiopian immigrant to Israel who consulted a traditional healer regarding her illness (rectal cancer) while also receiving chemotherapy. The traditional healer concluded the main cause of the illness to be a ganal or Satan occupying the woman's body. Another patient, a Tunisian immigrant to Israel, believed that his colorectal cancer was caused by a curse his sister had placed on the family ten years earlier. Imbalance of inner forces as a cause of illness is a belief held by many cultures across Asia, India, Spain and Latin America (Galanti, 1991; Hamilton, 1996). In Asia these counterbalancing forces are known as yin and yang. Yin is 'the receptive, recessive, submissive, and hidden background force represented by the female and earth' whereas yang is the 'creative, forward, dominating, and manifest force represented by the male and heaven' (Chan, 1992, p. 187). Illness or disease is believed to be caused by a disturbed balance between these forces. In general, treatment aims to return the body to equilibrium. For example, excessive yin (which is considered to produce cold, darkness, and sadness) is treated with foods, herbs, or other techniques considered to possess yang (warmth, light, and fullness).

Beliefs about the causes of illness or disability may have a significant impact on the patient's or parent's expectations about what can be done to treat or manage the condition. In any culture, whether illness and disability are regarded from a biomedical or traditional perspective, it will be expected that the treatment matches the perceived cause of the problem. If patients believe their illness to be caused by a bacterial infection, they will probably expect to be treated with antibiotics. If patients believe their illness to be caused by divine punishment for sins, they may expect penance to alleviate the problem. For example, the Tunisian patient suffering from colorectal cancer, as previously described, believed that his sister's blessing would cure his illness, removing the curse she had placed on the family ten years before. The Ethiopian woman suffering from rectal cancer used herbal medicines and daily visits to cold healing waters in an attempt to force the ganal from her body (Delbar, 1999).

Offering a treatment approach that does not reflect the perceived cause of illness/disability may result in feelings of dissatisfaction for the patient/family, non-compliance, and poor treatment outcomes. Thus, it is important for health professionals to acknowledge the patient's beliefs while explaining the unfamiliar treatment approach in a way that reflects their conceptual framework. Providing information to help the patient or parent understand the recommended assessment or treatment technique is essential and is best done with the assistance of a trained interpreter, if required, translated written material, and liaison with community leaders or community representatives who have experienced the recommended treatment approach. See, for example, Chan (1992, pp. 226-7) for a detailed case study of a family of a child with autism, for further information on these assessment and treatment considerations.

It is crucial to understand that, although a range of biomedical and traditional perceptions of illness have been presented, it should not be assumed that every individual from a given culture will respond to illness in exactly the same way. We have already seen how many factors influence a person's culture, including upbringing, education, peer relationships, employment, and so on. Each individual from a given culture will assume the beliefs, values, attitudes, and behaviours of the broader cultural context to varying degrees. It would be impossible to provide a checklist of 'do' and 'don't' rules for interacting with an indigenous American patient, a Japanese patient, a Russian patient, or a Turkish patient, for example. Acculturation refers to the process of cultural transition that occurs when an individual enters a new cultural context. An example of an individual entering a new cultural context would be a Vietnamese family migrating to North America. However, acculturation is not limited to new immigrants. Second- and even third-generation migrants who have remained within a relatively tight cultural community may enter a new cultural context when attending school or beginning employment, for example. Acculturation is a process, not an immediate response to the new cultural context, and the stage of acculturation assumed by patients will certainly influence their cultural makeup. An individual may move from total rejection of the new culture and immersion in their own culture to acceptance of both cultures and the ability to competently switch between cultures as required (with a variety of stages in between). It is even possible for members of the one family to assume different stages of the acculturation process. This process of cultural transition will ultimately influence the degree to which a patient identifies with their traditional cultural beliefs, including perceptions of illness and expectations about treatment. In any intercultural encounter it is important to be aware of potential differences in communication styles and behaviour so that miscommunications can be effectively and efficiently identified and repaired. At the same time it is vitally important to explore the patient's individual attitudes and beliefs, especially in relation to health care, illness, and treatment expectations.

Scott (1997) suggests that in any health-care context it is important to establish a 'cultural construct of clinical reality' (p. 179) to determine the patient's beliefs, views, attitudes and expectations about health and illness. She lists a variety of questions that can be used to facilitate clinical discussion, in order to gain a better insight into the patient's perceptions of their illness. For example:

- What do you think has caused you to be sick?
- Why do you think your sickness started when it did?

- What do you think your sickness does to you? How does it work?
- How sick are you?
- Do you think you are going to be sick for a long time? Or do you think you will get better soon?
- Will you get better on your own?
- Has anyone else you know ever had the same problem?
- What kind of treatment do you think you need?
- What are the most important results you hope to get from treatment?
- What are the major problems this illness has caused you – at home and other places?
- What do you fear most about what is going on?

MacLachlan (1997) proposed a method for 'understanding a person's inner experience' in relation to perceptions of illness and expected treatments (p. 62). In its most simple form the Problem Portrait Technique uses the patient's own description of the presenting problem and maps the various causes attributed to it. After identifying their own perceptions of the cause of their illness, MacLachlan suggests that patients should be encouraged to identify the perceptions of significant others (for example parent, sibling, other relation, friend, community group). In this way, patients may describe some causes which they did not identify from their own reflection, but which still exert an influence over their perception of the illness. Patients then rate each cause in terms of their perception of its relative strength. This allows the clinician to see what causes the patient really identifies with. Finally, for each cause the patient is asked to describe the appropriate treatment. These treatments are also rated according to the patient's perception of each treatment's relative strength. Now the clinician is able to see which causes patients identify with and which treatments they expect to work. MacLachlan suggests using a visual web of concentric circles to map causes, treatments, and ratings (along radii), with the patient's description of the problem at the centre.

Figure 3.1 shows a hypothetical Problem Portrait for stuttering. In this example, the patient has identified physical problems and punishment as causal factors. He identified emotional problems and fate as common causal beliefs within his cultural group. Finally, he identified laziness as a cause, reflecting the belief of his family, especially his parents. Consequential treatments for each causal factor were listed as exercises (physical problem), prayer and offerings (punishment), counselling (emotional disturbance), no treatment (fate), and trying harder (laziness). The patient was then asked to rate his relative belief in each of the causes and treatments identified. These were then mapped onto the Problem Portrait diagram, with causes represented in the inner circle and treatments in the outer circle.

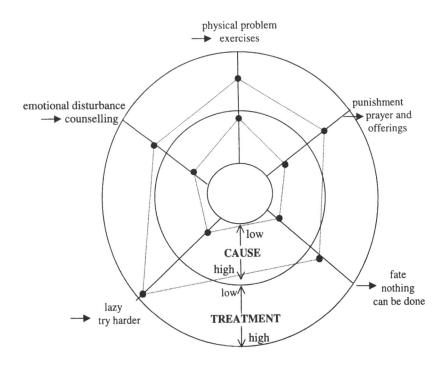

Figure 3.1. The Problem Portrait Technique (MacLachlan, 1997) showing perceived causes of and expected treatments for stuttering.

This hypothetical diagram illustrates the potential discrepancy between a patient's belief in causes and consequential treatments. For example, the patient has given a relatively low rating to *laziness* as a cause, but a relatively high rating to its consequential treatment, *trying harder*. Similarly, the patient has given a relatively high rating to *physical problem* as a cause, but a lower rating to its consequential treatment, *exercises*. So, how does this influence clinical decisions for effective and appropriate management planning? Helping the patient to identify perceived causes and treatments for their communication difficulties will raise your awareness of their clinical reality and help you to plan intervention with open consideration of the patient's perspective. In the example above, the patient's strong belief that the stuttering is caused by a physical problem that can be successfully treated by trying harder could be used to your advantage in the clinical context. Informing the patient about current theories on the causes of stuttering and choosing a treatment approach based on repeated practice in structured linguistic contexts, such as an Extended Length of Utterance approach (Costello Ingham, 1993), may be more acceptable to the patient than an approach based on modification of speech patterns, for example. Modification of speech patterns may be more acceptable when the patient places a higher emphasis on stuttering as a physical problem. The important point is choosing an approach that is as congruent as possible with patients' perception of their communication difficulty and their expectations of treatment. Implementing a treatment approach that contrasts with the patient's perceptions and expectations may adversely affect patient/family compliance, attendance, and ultimately, progress.

MacLachlan acknowledges that a detailed Problem Portrait, such as the one for stuttering, is the 'Rolls Royce version' (p. 71). Time restraints and language barriers may prohibit such a thorough analysis. Yet, even when a simplified version is completed (perhaps based on only two or three causes/treatments, looking at treatments only, or just analysing the patient's perspective), MacLachlan argues that 'the orientation adopted through using the technique should enhance the quality of clinical assessment and therefore the efficacy of the treatment' (p. 71). Thus, it may be worth the extra time to get some idea of the patient's perspective, however simplified the analysis may be.

Making intercultural health care work

Wells (1995) suggests that in every health-care context there are at least three cultures involved — the personal culture of the clinician, the personal culture of the patient, and the culture of the health-care system. Often in intercultural contacts these are vastly different, and disregard for these differences may only result in communication breakdown, feelings of dissatisfaction, poor outcomes, non-compliance, and perhaps even misdiagnosis. Kanitsaki (1993) reports a case where a middle-aged Hungarian woman was taken to an emergency department by her daughter (a registered psychiatric nurse) because of persistent severe headaches and personality change over the past five years. The daughter was very anxious and keen for her mother to receive a thorough medical examination. There had not been any prior medical assessment performed, despite numerous consultations. However, after reviewing the patient's medical record, with the numerous accounts of past visits to the emergency department, the attending doctor documented the cause of illness as 'ethnic head' and 'menopausal syndrome'. The woman was discharged with a prescription for paracetamol [Tylenol] tablets and instructions to return to her family doctor. As she left the hospital, the woman suffered from a grand mal seizure. The attending doctor then ordered a CAT scan, which revealed a slow-growing frontal lobe brain tumour. The woman died two weeks later. *Ethnic head* is not a medically recognized diagnosis and illustrates the attending doctor's gross misjudgement of the patient's presenting symptoms and behaviours. Culture influences the way patients react to illness and the way they behave in the sick role. The attending doctor in the above scenario has demonstrated a lack of respect for cultural differences. The doctor has neglected to consider alternate interpretations to the patient's behaviour and has judged her according to personal stereotypes and attitudes — behaviour reflecting certainty orientation and narrow categorization. In this case the false negative judgement resulted in the worst outcome.

Intercultural health care encompasses all aspects of the health-care routine, including greetings, leave taking, interview style, question types, examination procedures, patient participation in decision making and management plans. Communicating with patients from diverse cultural backgrounds requires sensitivity towards those behavioural and linguistic interaction patterns that are influenced by culture, for example, non-verbal communication, politeness routines, use of silence, attitude towards direct questioning, language styles (for example, linear versus circular), and perceptions of illness and disability. When working with culturally diverse patients it is important to recognize the road to cultural competence and plan professional practices within an intercultural framework. The following list offers some considerations in providing a culturally focused approach to health care.

Considerations in providing a culturally focused approach to health care

- Be aware of the possibility of alternate interpretations, even if you are not sure what those alternates are. That is, be uncertainty oriented.
- Avoid judging the patient according to your own culturally biased stereotypes, beliefs, values, and perceptions. That is, be a broad categorizer.
- Be aware of your personal culture and professional culture and consider the way these influence your behaviours and communication styles.
- Maintain your motivation to culture learn since all cultures are dynamic and will inevitably change over time and with the force of external influences, such as contact with other cultural groups.
- Liaise with community leaders in each cultural group to discuss your services and determine strategies for improved and more equitable practice.
- Be aware of your own limitations in working with culturally diverse populations — know when to seek help and where to find it.
- Determine the patient's views and perceptions of illness and disability and their expectations of you — that is, determine their clinical reality.

- Be aware that the interview style with which you are comfortable may not be culturally appropriate or relevant to your patient — look for signs of misunderstanding.
- Acknowledge the patients' perspective, listen to their concerns and provide information within their conceptual framework.

CHAPTER 4

Intercultural speech-language pathology

Speech-language pathology (SLP) is a relatively modern discipline stemming from a biomedical approach to health care. It is culture bound — that is, it is bound to the culture of biomedical health care. Thus, the concept of SLP is foreign in many cultural groups around the world. In the last chapter we looked at perceptions of illness and disability from a cultural perspective and found that the way people respond to illness/disability and the cause they attribute to illness/disability is often deeply rooted in cultural beliefs. The same cultural variability applies to perceptions of communication disorders and, therefore, perceptions of assessment and treatment procedures. In recent years, with an increasing focus on the health-care needs of patients from diverse cultural backgrounds, there has been a push to make health-care services more equitable and accessible to all cultural groups.

Speech-language pathology is a complex field of health care. We deal with a large variety of communication and swallowing disorders in patients from birth to the elderly. Often there is coexisting illness or disability that further impacts on the patient's communication or swallowing difficulty; and often there is a real potential for the disorder to negatively impact on other aspects of the patient's life, such as social and work function, or academic performance. We often work in centres with long waiting lists and limited resources (human and material) and are frequently challenged to reduce waiting times and increase patient throughput. Many families are familiar with this type of health reform strategy and seem to deal with changes to service delivery without significant difficulty. However, changes such as an increase in consultative services, home programming, limited sessions, and use of aides may only make SLP more alien and more incongruent to some patients from diverse cultural backgrounds.

An intercultural look at SLP sessions

Read through the following session descriptions and try to identify any aspects that may be subject to intercultural variation. The first scenario describes a paediatric assessment session. The second scenario describes an adult treatment session.

Scenario 1 — paediatric assessment

Your next appointment is 10:15 a.m. You walk out to the waiting area and see two children playing with toys while mother, father, and grandmother wait close by. You introduce yourself by your full name and explain that you are the speech-language pathologist seeing Joseph today. You suggest that it may be best if someone stays out with Joseph's brother, so he can play without disturbing the assessment, and because your office is fairly small. You assume that this is why the grandmother has come along. Mum and dad stand to follow you in to your office as you gently steer Joseph in the right direction with a guiding hand on his head.

Inside your office you offer Joseph some toys to play with and invite his parents to sit down. You sit opposite the parents and begin your assessment session by interviewing them about Joseph's development, past medical history, hearing history, school performance, their concerns, and his teacher's concerns. With the interview complete, you briefly explain the procedure for the assessment. You suggest that the mother or father move onto the floor with Joseph to facilitate a conversational sample that will give you an insight into his communication skills. Once you have an adequate conversational sample, you ask Joseph to join you at the table for some formal assessment procedures. You complete a more detailed phonological assessment and an expressive language screening. At the end of the assessment you praise Joseph extensively for working so hard and reward him with a sticker and stamp. He plays freely on the floor again while you speak with his parents about the results of the assessment and discuss options for treatment. You explain that Joseph presents with a moderate communication disorder that will require intervention. He will have to go on another waiting list for individual therapy but you suggest they attend a language group and work on an artic-ulation home programme until individual therapy is available.

This scenario may describe the type of session with which you are familiar and comfortable. Yet, in an encounter with a family from a cultural background different to your own, this session may present many problems. Let's now look at some of these issues.

'Your next appointment is 10:15 a.m. You walk out to the waiting area and see two children playing . . .'

The family has arrived for the appointment on time (or perhaps early). In a time-driven society, we expect patients/customers/visitors to arrive on time.

We often leave little room for tardiness before beginning to feel frustrated and annoyed. Punctuality is valued and expected. However, time orientation is influenced by culture. Galanti (1991) suggests that present time-oriented cultures believe that the future will arrive in its own time, and therefore it is impossible to be late. Arriving at 11:00 a.m., or later, for a 10:15 a.m. appointment would not be considered late. In a busy SLP clinic, however, it is difficult to allow for variations in time orientation. With consecutive patients, scheduled meetings, school visits, family conferences, and ward rounds, there is little opportunity to 'fit in' appointments whenever the patient arrives unscheduled. Planning for the possibility that the scheduled appointment time may not be understood as the only appointment time, is necessary. Appointment cards, phone bookings, reminder calls, may need to reinforce the importance of arriving as close to the appointment time as possible. For larger patient numbers, drop-in days may be a more useful and successful service delivery option.

'You assume that this is why the grandmother has come along.'

Cultural groups can be described as individualist or collectivist. Individualist cultures place more value on self-achievements and independence, and exist within the framework of the immediate family. Nuclear families operate independently, with the parents being the dominant carers for children. Collectivist cultures, in contrast, place greater value on group achievements and group membership, and exist within the framework of the extended family and community group. Child rearing is often shared among members of the family or community group, extending to grandparents, aunts, or neighbours. The extended family often live together, or at least close by, so that the mother may not act as the dominant carer, especially when there are other life stresses present. In this case, the grandparent, aunt, or neighbour, may have the most information about the child's development, achievements and difficulties. Thus, it cannot be assumed that the parents will be the greatest source of information. The primary carer needs to be identified as soon as possible, perhaps at the time of referral, so that they can attend the appointment to assist with the interview, or to hear about management strategies. In the above example, the grandmother may share the role of primary carer with the mother, or be the dominant carer instead of the mother. It may be more appropriate for the father to wait outside with the second son while you interview Joseph's mother and grandmother.

'. . . you gently steer Joseph in the right direction with a guiding hand on his head.'

In a review of the literature, Singelis (1994) found that non-verbal communication was reported to account for between 65% and 93% of total communication. Despite this variation, it is clear that non-verbal communication plays a very important role in conveying meaning. Non-verbal behaviours, such as eye contact, use of silence, gesture, and physical contact can convey vastly different meanings across cultures. Although, in the above example, the clinician may have touched the child's head in a friendly gesture, some cultural groups see this behaviour in a very different way. Chan (1992) reports that some Asian cultural groups, such as Cambodians, Lao, and some Buddhists believe touching a child's (or adult's) head to be threatening or offensive because of the strong spiritual belief that the head is the most sacred part of the body.

'You sit opposite the parents . . .'

Eye contact is a non-verbal behaviour able to convey strong meanings in any communicative interaction. The value placed on eye contact and knowledge of appropriate forms and uses will vary considerably across cultures. In the culture with which I am familiar, eye contact is an expected part of communicative exchange. When the listener maintains direct eye contact with the speaker, he or she is signalling interest in what is being said. In cultures where this belief is held, speakers often sit or stand so that they are able to achieve good eye contact. Often, opposite each other. In many cultures where direct eye contact signals anger, hostility, or invasion, it is more appropriate for the communicative partners to position themselves in a way where direct eye contact is less achievable. Often, this is adjacent to each other. A person's level of comfort can be significantly reduced in a communicative exchange when their social-behavioural rules are violated.

'. . . interviewing them about Joseph's development, past medical history, hearing history, school performance, their concerns, and his teacher's concerns.'

As SLPs, we are concerned about the relationship between a patient's developmental/medical history and the presenting communication disorder. In paediatric case history interviews we would be interested in the mother's pregnancy, labour and birth information, the child's early developmental milestones, relevant illnesses or hospitalizations, language and social experiences including child-rearing practices, and so on. Families that are familiar with a biomedical approach to health-care services may expect these questions to be asked without the need for explanation, circumlocution, or extended lead-up talk. However, in some cultures it is considered rude and intrusive to ask questions of a personal nature, such as pregnancy and birth, too soon in the interview. In other cultures, it is acceptable to ask these questions when there is a sharing of information between the patient/family and professional. In such cases, the patient/carer may ask personal questions of the SLP, such as 'what is your background?', 'where do you live?', 'How long have you lived here?', 'Are you married?', 'How many children do you have?', and so on. This type of exchange may be expected as part of the routine of information gathering.

'You suggest that the mother or father move onto the floor with Joseph to facilitate a conversational sample . . .'

Parents may participate in free play with their children, without question, when they believe and engage in parent–child play as part of their child-rearing strategy. However, not all families believe that parents and children should interact at this level. Play, and its associated chatter, may be left to siblings, cousins and friends, but not adults. Where the goal of free play is to gather a conversational sample for an informal analysis of language, voice, phonology, or fluency, comfortable and natural interaction is paramount. Parents who do not actively engage in parent–child play at home are unlikely to feel comfortable performing this in a clinic, in front of an observing clinician. The situation would be unfamiliar to both the parent and child, and may result in an inadequate sample for assessment purposes. If the child is unfamiliar with adult–child play or has a strong belief in respecting elders and authority figures, the SLP may also gain little from attempts to engage the child in play. Lack of awareness of the cultural influence on a child's behaviour in interaction with an adult may result in descriptions like *passive communicator, poor pragmatic skills, or demonstrates poor eye contact, topic initiation and topic maintenance* when, in fact, these behaviours are contextually appropriate in that child's culture. In the above case scenario, it may be more useful to observe Joseph and his brother in free play. If siblings or other children are not present during the session, it may be necessary to schedule another appointment when siblings, cousins, or friends can attend, conduct a home visit, or, if appropriate, a school visit. In most cases, thorough assessment of patients from culturally and linguistically diverse backgrounds will require more than one appointment. Indeed, as will be discussed in later chapters, dynamic assessment over time is an effective culturally focused tool. Informal assessment plans for the first session may be replaced with an expanded parent interview, perhaps encompassing detailed information about concerns and perceptions (a Problem Portrait could be completed for cause — see Chapter 3 for a discussion of this approach), language exposures and patterns of use for bilingual children, and so on. Similarly, other, more structured assessment tasks relying on patient–clinician interaction could be completed. When using siblings or friends in the clinic setting it is important to recreate a naturalistic environment that would be familiar and comfortable to the children, including culturally appropriate games, activities, and materials. If conducting a home visit it will be important to identify any additional cultural considerations, such as removing shoes at the door, where to sit, how to sit, accepting tea, and so on.

'. . . you ask Joseph to join you at the table for some formal assessment procedures.'

Before conducting a formal assessment battery, it is important to consider the child's experience with testing formats. If the child is not yet attending school, the structured question–answer technique may be very foreign. In addition, formal assessment tools are often standardized on a narrow population, such as middle-class, Anglo-European children. It can almost be assumed that these children have had similar cultural, social, and educational experiences. They represent the standards for average, above average, and below average that can be expected in the target cultural group. Yet, not all children we assess will fall into such a narrow population focus. Test stimuli, including materials, pictures, objects, and questions, as well as testing procedures and scoring criteria can vary considerably in their application to different cultural groups. Even across what we would expect to be very similar cultural groups there can be significant variation in the cultural appropriateness of test stimuli. Tests that are standardized on a narrow population set may restrict performance diversity and result in a limited and possibly biased response pool. Prescribed scoring techniques may not allow for non-standard responses and may result in false negative outcomes for the patient. The responsibility falls on the clinician to interpret test results descriptively and with caution. A patient's poor test performance may be the result of unfamiliarity with testing procedures or items as opposed to specific speech or language difficulty. Standardized assessment and scoring techniques are discussed in greater detail in Chapter 5.

'You complete a more detailed phonological assessment and an expressive language screening.'

When assessing children from diverse cultural backgrounds, it is important to consider the phonological and linguistic structure of the child's home language, if that is not English, as well as their exposure to and experience with English. Applying the phonological and morpho-syntactic rules of your own language to the child's sample may provide you with false-negative information. It may be appropriate to say that a child has a limited command of the phonological and morpho-syntactic features of English and therefore demonstrates a functional incompetence in English-language contexts. However, it may be inappropriate to label the child as speech or language disordered. For example, in Chinese languages, such as Mandarin, there are no digraphs, so that *something* may be pronounced as *somesing* (Chan, 1992). There are only two final consonants used in Mandarin (*n* and *ng*) and seven in Cantonese (*m*, *n*, *ng*, *p*, *t*, *k*, and *glottal stop*) so that it may be appropriate for a child with limited English-language experience to demonstrate difficulty with final consonants (Cheng, 1993). Morpho-syntactically, there are no gender pronouns, plurals, or tense markers. These features are denoted contextually or by the addition of whole words within a sentence (Chan, 1992). Difficulty with the phonological, morphological, and syntactic features of English may be indicative of speech/language difference as opposed to speech/language disorder.

'At the end of the assessment you praise Joseph extensively for working so hard and reward him with a sticker and stamp.'

Verbal praise and material reinforcement are considered appropriate in some cultures. Speech-language pathologists may use verbal praise and material reinforcers, such as stickers, stamps, or a turn at a game, to reward good behaviour, attention, and performance, or to encourage continued motivation and concentration. Children from cultures where praise and rewards are a common feature of behaviour management and child-rearing practices are likely to respond positively. In contrast to this, some cultures believe that success will be achieved only if the child tries hard enough, and hard work is, therefore, expected. Praise and rewards may be seen as inappropriate and may not have the same impact on the child.

'You explain that Joseph presents with a moderate communication disorder . . .'

A child who presents with similar communication difficulties across both languages may, indeed, have a traditional communication disorder. However, it is important to consider the child's language exposures and experiences before analysing speech and language samples. While it is not necessarily important to distinguish between a communication disorder as opposed to a difficulty due to speech or language difference, it is important to determine the child's communication competence in different situational contexts. Thus, the decision to provide treatment can be based on the more functional measure of competence rather than the subjective presence of a disorder. This issue is explored in further detail later in Chapter 5.

'. . . you suggest they attend a language group and work on an articulation home programme . . .'

With increasing pressure on SLP services to provide treatment to more and more patients with fewer resources, waiting lists are inevitable and alternative service delivery models have to be employed. Home programmes and group therapy are commonly used and are often effective management strategies. Yet, there can be considerable variance in the perceived value of group therapy or compliance with home programmes within the dominant cultural group. Thus, variation across cultural groups should be expected. Some families may expect the speech-language pathologist to provide an immediate answer to the child's communication difficulty — a fast and effective treatment — not the prospect of long-term intervention, especially not one that is administered by the family. Some families may be reluctant to attend or participate in group therapy for fear of embarrassment in front of other parents, perhaps feeling that their parenting skills are on display. Group therapy activities will need to be carefully selected, considering cultural variation in parenting techniques, approaches to play, attitude towards reinforcement, familiarity with songs, stories, toys, materials, and so on. Before offering management options, it would be valuable to identify the family's expectations regarding treatment (including approach, procedures, outcomes, and time frame) and their willingness to be involved in the therapy.

Let us now look at another scenario, this time involving an adult patient in a hospital-based therapy session.

Scenario 2 — adult therapy session

You enter the hospital room to find your patient reclining in bed, his wife sitting in the chair beside him. You cheerfully greet them both and casually chat about the day. You explain that you are here to go through some more therapy exercises. You help your patient sit up in the bed and prop him upright with another pillow. You sit in another seat next to the bed and ask the patient if he has noticed any changes in his communication since starting therapy. You then ask his wife if she has noticed any changes. When you ask how they are going with the exercises you left for them to practise twice a day, they indicate no problems. You suggest they continue practising them twice a day. You move on to work on your patient's word retrieval. You use object flash cards to elicit spontaneous labelling. When he has difficulty you provide a semantic cue followed by a phonemic cue, if needed, to prompt word retrieval. Your patient describes his frustration at not being able to get the words out and you are able to counsel him with regard to how the stroke has affected his speech using a neuroanatomical and cognitive-neuropsychological explanation. You explain the rationale for the therapy activity based on these models and suggest a long road to recovery with the need for regular practise. However, his obvious frustration leads you to consider the option of an augmentative communication system. You decide to discuss this with your patient and his wife. Your patient is keen for an augmentative communication system to help communicate with medical and nursing staff when his wife is not there. As he is still having difficulty reading and writing words, you suggest a picture communication system. You spend the remainder of the session discussing his communicative needs before leaving to prepare the communication system.

This scenario may, again, describe the type of session with which you are familiar and comfortable. Yet, it also presents many potential problems when it describes an encounter with a patient from a cultural background different from your own.

'You explain that you are here to go through some more therapy exercises.'

In Australia, England, America, and Europe, for example, women in professional practice are common. Such women would expect to be treated fairly and equally and command the same respect in their jobs as their male counterparts. However, in more traditional cultures, women may not be ascribed the same degree of respect or equality, especially by men. A female speech-language pathologist treating a male patient may find that the patient holds little respect for her professional knowledge or competence. The patient may not express this directly. Instead, it may be conveyed through non-compliance or reluctance to offer information. This, however, is a situation that cannot always be changed. A female SLP is a female SLP and, unless she has a male colleague who is able to take on the case, she must continue to provide appropriate management for her patient. It may help to liaise with community leaders, ethnic health workers, interpreters, or other experts in cross-gender cultural differences to identify useful methods for establishing a more effective relationship with the patient.

'You help your patient sit up in the bed and prop him upright with another pillow.'

Cultural attitudes towards gender and age differences can impact heavily on a patient's comfort with physical assistance. The patient may prefer to manage on their own or obtain their wife's assistance rather than the assistance of a younger, female SLP.

'You then ask his wife if she has noticed any changes.'

Some cultures are vertically structured, maintaining a strong belief in male dominance. Asking the wife her opinion of her husband's speech may place the husband in an embarrassing situation, causing loss of face. In response to this, the wife may exaggerate her husband's abilities so that he appears better. The SLP may then find that s/he has unreliable information, and has managed to inadvertently embarrass the patient and his wife.

'When you ask how they are going with the exercises you left for them to practise twice a day, they indicate no problems.'

Many patients, from cultures that believe in maintaining interpersonal harmony, will not admit difficulty for fear of losing face or further troubling the SLP. Face-saving is important. The patient may prefer to imply that everything is OK rather than admit a problem and risk losing face. To confirm whether or not the patient is having trouble, it may be better to try one (or more) of the following approaches:

* Ask that he demonstrate or explain what he has been doing — care needs to be taken with this approach as some patients may feel it devalues their independence and integrity.
* Encourage further discussion by offering examples of common difficulties patients have with practice exercises (for example, time restraints; lack of adequate equipment; environmental disruptions such as noise, interruptions; physical difficulty with the activity; lack of clinician's model, and so on).
* Spend the first few minutes of the session revising the practice activity together — check for any difficulties, confusion, or discomfort/frustration — this revision can be completed routinely as a planned therapy goal for each session.

'You use object flash cards to elicit spontaneous labelling.'

The purpose and rationale for such an activity may not be understood. Some patients may expect a more functional approach or view the therapy activity as baby-like. This attitude may also be found in any patient, regardless of culture. However, patients who are more familiar with traditional methods of healing may expect therapy to reflect their beliefs. Object flash cards may be as foreign to them as folk-healing remedies are to you. It is always important, then, to be aware of the patient's understanding of the problem, its cause, nature, appropriate treatment, and expected outcome. Scott's questions for developing a cultural construct of clinical reality (1997) can be modified to elicit information about specific communication or swallowing problems. This is expanded on later in this chapter.

'When he has difficulty you provide a semantic cue followed by a phonemic cue, if needed, to prompt word retrieval.'

In addition to cultural variability in expectations about treatment approaches, there will also be the potential for cultural bias in the stimuli items used during assessment or treatment sessions. Object flash cards may include items with which patients are not familiar, or that they do not know by name, especially if they have maintained a more traditional existence, within a tight cultural community. Inability to name the object may reflect lack of knowledge rather than difficulties with word retrieval. It can be useful to go through the cards first to identify any with which the patient is unfamiliar.

'Your patient describes his frustration . . .'

Describing frustration is similar to admitting difficulty and may result in loss of face. Describing frustration may also be emotionally charged. Patients from cultures that hold the belief that strong emotions should not be demonstrated in public may choose to remain silent in the face of frustration. In addition, frustration may be exhibited in other, less obvious ways, such as reluctance to continue, non-compliance, smiling or laughing. Not recognizing a patient's frustrations may mean that opportunities to improve the management approach may be missed. The SLP may not see that counselling is needed or that the management approach needs to be modified.

'. . . you are able to counsel him with regard to how the stroke has affected his speech using a neuroanatomical and cognitive-neuropsychological explanation.'

Following a biomedical model, SLPs often explain communication disorders following stroke in terms of site of lesion, brain function, and/or a breakdown along a neuropsychological pathway, for example from word selection to speech execution. This scientific model relies heavily on an understanding of the brain as a complex organ, made up of nerve cells, blood vessels, and nerve fibre tracts, which has control over many mental, motor, and sensory activities. Patients from cultures that believe in a biomedical model of health and illness are likely to accept a neuroanatomical or neuropsychological explanation, although they may not fully understand it. Patients from cultures which view health and illness in a more traditional light, perhaps attributing illness to punishment from angry spirits or an imbalance of inner forces, such as yin and yang, are less likely to accept the biomedical explanation (although they may not indicate this). It is important to respect the patient's beliefs and, where possible, offer explanations within the patient's conceptual framework.

'... *his obvious frustration leads you to consider the option of an augmentative communication system.*'

Augmentative communication systems are usually conspicuous and identify the patient as having a disability. However, some patients may accept the suggestion enthusiastically, seeing the opportunity to improve and expand their communication, while others fear that the system will label them as disabled. This variation occurs within cultures as well as across cultures. Patients from more traditional cultures may have strong beliefs that disability should be hidden, that they should not be a burden on their family, and that they should accept whatever outcome as fate. Patients with these beliefs may be reluctant to use an augmentative communication system, especially if it is bulky and conspicuous.

'... *you suggest a picture communication system.*'

As with assessment and therapy stimuli, picture systems can be subject to cultural bias. It is important to select pictures that reflect the patient's experiences. If the patient only uses chopsticks, or a spoon and fork, avoid using a picture of a knife and fork. Pictures of food should be culturally relevant, such as a bowl of rice instead of a hamburger to represent *dinner.* Where possible use real pictures of people, such as family members and significant others. Pictures of daily activities should be realistic, reflecting the patient's knowledge and experiences. Pictures that have a strong cultural bias and may not, therefore, be familiar to people outside the patient's cultural reality, should also include a written word or description.

Attitudes towards communication disorders

In 1992, Linda Bebout and Bradford Arthur published a paper investigating cultural influences on attitudes towards various communication disorders. In their research project, they surveyed 166 students across two universities in the US and Canada. The students were all English speaking but identified themselves as either North American/Canadian, Chinese, Southeast Asian, Japanese, Malaysian, Taiwanese, Singaporean, or Hispanic. The questionnaire survey looked at attitudes towards four communication disorders — severe adult stuttering, the speech of the hearing impaired, cleft palate, and misarticulation in older children. For each of the disorders, the survey asked respondents to rate their opinion on twelve statements relating to the perceived cause of the disorder, the family/community's attitude towards the person, and the desirability of the person seeking help.

Of most interest to SLPs is the clear distinction between North American/Canadian subjects and foreign-born subjects in their opinion that the person could improve their speech if they tried hard enough. Across all disorder types there was a significant difference in opinion, with foreign-born subjects more likely to believe that the communication disorder could be improved if the person tried hard enough. People who believe this may, therefore, be less likely to seek intervention for themselves or their child. If intervention is sought, there may be the expectation that the treatment will be successful if the patient tries his or her hardest. In the treatment of stuttering, a behavioural approach, wherein fluent speech is praised, may not be accepted by families who expect their children to try harder, and therefore should not need to be praised. Significant difference was also found across the four disorder types in opinion about emotional stability. Foreign-born subjects were more likely to perceive the person with a communication disorder as emotionally disturbed. In assuming a common relationship between communication disorders and emotional disturbance, patients or their families may not seek medical advice or intervention for the emotional problem. Unresolved and untreated emotional problems relating to the communication disorder can have a negative impact on the patient's subsequent progress in and compliance with treatment.

Perceptions about the cause, nature, and treatment of communication disorders are strongly influenced by culture. A more traditional understanding of the cause of the disorder (for example, broken traditions, punishment by fate or God, improper diet or broken taboos) will foster more traditional expectations about treatment. If intervention is sought it will be important to identify the patient/family's perceptions and expectations through establishing their cultural construct of clinical reality. The list of questions from Scott (1997, p. 179) can be modified to relate more specifically to communication disorders:

- What do you think has caused your/your child's communication disorder?
- Why do you think your/your child's communication disorder started when it did?
- What effect does the communication disorder have on you/your child? On your family?
- How severe is your/your child's communication disorder?
- Do you think the communication disorder will be with you/your child for a long time? Or do you think it will go away soon?

- Will the problem get better on its own?
- Has anyone else you know ever had the same problem?
- What kind of treatment do you think is needed?
- What do you expect treatment to do for you/your child?
- Do you fear anything about your/your child's communication disorder? What do you fear?

In each question an appropriate communication (or swallowing) problem should be substituted for *communication disorder*. For example, *what do you think has caused your child's speech problem?* Understanding the patient/family's reality will reduce the risk of conflict and will help the SLP identify appropriate management strategies, such as the ones listed below:

- Align the treatment approach with the family's perceptions and expectations (for example, use of praise and rewards may be less accepted or less effective when patients are expected to try their hardest).
- Provide counselling regarding the communication disorder within the patient/family's conceptual understanding (for example, suggesting that the communication disorder is an effect of the stroke, while perhaps acknowledging the patient's belief that the stroke was punishment for past sins — in this way it may still be possible to work from a neuroanatomical explanation for the communication impairment while respecting the patient's traditional beliefs).
- Establish goals that address the patient/family's areas of concern regarding the effect of the communication disorder and perceived severity. Clinical severity may not match personal or cultural perceptions. Thus, a clinically mild disorder may be perceived as a great problem. For patients with multiple disorders, it may be necessary to address a mild problem before or at the same time as a more clinically severe disorder.
- Address unrealistic expectations regarding treatment by providing information and examples to which the patient can relate. For example, provide translated information, access to support groups within their cultural community (where available), contact with other patients/families who have been through a similar experience, liaise with community leaders and offer information regarding speech-language pathology and specific communication disorders, and so on.

Activity 4.1

Reflect on a typical assessment and treatment session you have performed and try to identify the communicative and social behaviours that have been influenced by your culture (it may help to watch a videotape of yourself). Which of these may have different meanings in other cultures or which may present potential barriers to the success of an intercultural speech-language pathology session?

In answering this question we need to consider the many ways in which culture can influence our own ways of being, behaving and communicating. Our work lives are by no means immune to this strong cultural influence. Our attitudes towards work practices, our ethics, behaviours, assessment and treatment approaches, communication styles, and so on are all vulnerable to the influence of our cultural heritage. Indeed, speech-language pathology as a profession is grounded in a distinct culture, reflecting a scientific model, so it follows that the approaches, procedures, and techniques that we traditionally use are based on that culture.

In reflecting on your own experiences in SLP sessions (assessment and treatment) you may have considered the following communicative and social behaviours that have been influenced by your cultural background:

Introduction style

- eye contact;
- direct language;
- use of names and titles (for example, Mrs, Mr);
- chat with patient/carer as part of introduction in waiting room;
- where you stand or sit in relation to the patient/carer;
- physical contact (for example, shaking hands, touching the patient on the arm);
- how you introduce yourself (first name or title plus surname, whether you provide any information about your qualifications and professional status, and so forth).

In the clinic room

- seating arrangements — for example, formal or informal, across a desk, in a circle, side-by-side;
- use of small talk before starting the session;
- sitting position — for example, cross legged, feet outstretched, arms folded or open.

Interview style

- use of note taking;
- eye contact;
- direct versus indirect questioning style;

- open versus closed questioning style;
- use of explanations regarding relevance of questions;
- body language — postures and gestures;
- facial expressions;
- who the questions are aimed at — for example, patient, wife, husband, mother, father.

Assessment/treatment

- explanation of procedures;
- physical contact with patient;
- feedback style;
- use of reinforcement/encouragement — verbal and/or material;
- seating arrangements;
- body language — postures, gestures, facial expressions;
- method of note taking, scoring.

Leave taking

- physical contact with patient/carer — for example, touching arm, head, shaking hands;
- use of small talk;
- facial expressions, gestures;
- use of humour;
- walking patient/carer out;
- language style — formal or informal register;
- use of first names or surname plus title.

You may have been able to identify further communicative and social behaviours pertinent to your own particular work style and work place. The ones I have listed above are fairly general and are probably typical in most SLP sessions. How you use each of the behaviours listed will depend on your culture and professional style. For instance, when greeting a child and parent in the waiting room at the start of a session, I may use first names for myself and the parent (for example, 'Hi Julie. I'm Kim. I'm the speech pathologist seeing Tommy today'). Here it is important to consider personal stylistic variation. I often feel comfortable using first names when the parent is the mother and of a similar age to myself. For older parents/grandparents or adult patients I use a more formal address (Mr/Mrs) until given permission to use a first name. Some SLPs may not feel comfortable using first names at all, regardless of the patient's/parent's age or gender. Following this I will often have some sort of chat with the child before moving into the room, as a way of introducing myself and helping them feel relaxed and comfortable with me. Whatever your approach, there is no right or wrong way of doing things — we will all use different methods depending on our professional style, which will be influenced by our social and professional cultures. Indeed, we will often change our behaviours to suit different clinical scenarios. The point to bear in mind, though, is that just as your clinical behaviours may differ from mine, your patient's expectations of your clinical and professional behaviours may also be very different. For example, your patient may expect you to behave in an authoritative professional manner, using a formal register, telling the patient information as opposed to promoting joint decision making, and so on. Your patient may expect you to identify the problem without questioning about symptoms or assessing skills. Physical touching, such as touching a patient on the arm as a sign of reassurance or encouragement, may be seen as totally inappropriate. Sitting on the floor with your legs extended and soles of your shoes pointing towards the patient or other family members may be considered extremely rude. Your patient may be more comfortable answering open-ended questions as opposed to closed questions or it may be the other way around. There are innumerable ways in which the social and communicative behaviours you use in a session can be interpreted differently by someone from a culture other than your own and they all present potential barriers to the success of a session if not considered in your preplanning and certainly during the session. It will be impossible for anyone to be aware of all the potential interpretations and expectations of every patient because people vary within cultures almost as much as they vary across cultures. Just as we observe the behaviours and communication styles of our patients in same culture/same language interactions and modify our behaviours accordingly, we must be even more aware within an intercultural interaction and strive to be broad categorizers and uncertainty oriented.

CHAPTER 5

Assessment and treatment approaches

The potential for cultural bias in assessment and treatment of communication disorders has already been touched on. This section aims to explore the nature and implications of cultural bias in greater detail.

Culturally focused assessment techniques

Most SLPs would be familiar with a range of formal standardized tests as well as informal assessment techniques. Formal assessment tools, as previously discussed, are often standardized on a very narrow population set, reflecting the dominant cultural group. Cultural bias in assessment procedures and stimuli is therefore a very real risk. The question–answer nature of many tests may be foreign or even threatening to some patients. Children taught to respect authority figures, such as doctors and teachers, may be reluctant to speak. Some question forms and linguistic concepts may be unfamiliar. Picture stimuli may reflect things with which the patient has had little or no experience. It is vitally important, then, for SLPs to carefully select assessment procedures and tools so that the most appropriate and useful information can be gathered from the patient. Disregard for cultural variation and the potential for cultural bias may result in wasted session time, poor outcomes, dissatisfaction, and the risk of basing diagnosis on unrealistic results. The following sections provide more detailed information on culturally focused assessment.

Functional scoring

If choosing to use a standardized assessment test, it is important to consider how you will score a non-standard response. Most assessment tests provide strict scoring criteria to help distinguish between patients who can and patients who can't produce the required response, due to some speech or language disorder. However, how do you account for patients who can't perform the task due to cultural difference, such as lack of exposure to or experience with the test item? By using the test's prescribed scoring criteria the SLP runs the risk of misdiagnosing the patient as communication disordered. It is a very black-and-white approach that neglects to consider what the patient is actually able to do. A culturally focused scoring method considers what the patient is able to do as opposed to what they are unable to do. Scoring is, therefore, subjective and qualitative. Your results take the form of a description rather than a numerical figure. For example, in assessing vocabulary, a child who responds to a picture of a thermometer by saying 'the nurse used it to see how hot I was when I was sick' would probably score zero using the test's prescribed scoring criteria. However, a functional scoring method recognizes that this child has provided a valuable insight into its linguistic abilities. Despite not knowing the actual label for 'thermometer', this child has demonstrated an understanding of the linguistic associations of the word. For 'thermometer' the child has given three linguistic elements — who can use a thermometer (nurse), when it is used (sick), and why it is used (hot). In addition, this child understands and expresses a comparative concept — the thermometer is not just used to see *if* you are hot, but to see *how* hot you really are. It should be clarified here that using standardized tests as a main component of assessment, even when scoring is modified, is not a recommended approach. Culturally focused assessment requires much greater evaluation and modification of assessment practices then just functional scoring. However, at times standardized tests may be used, in entirety or in part, as a small part of a much greater ethnographic assessment process. The key point to remember is whenever using a standardized test, responses should be interpreted descriptively using modified scoring techniques to highlight what linguistic features the patient has while considering alternate reasons for the patient's poor performance. Even tests which have been translated or designed specifically for bilingual patient populations should be carefully examined regarding validity for individual patients given the diversity within cultural and language groups. A more detailed discussion of available translated English-language and bilingual assessment tools is offered later in this chapter.

Informal assessment

Informal assessment approaches can be tailored to suit each individual patient. Culturally appropriate materials and procedures can be employed, and a variety of settings and communicative partners used. For this reason, informal assessment methods are likely to provide more realistic information than standardized testing. The assessment situation should be as naturalistic as possible, with low patient anxiety and high motivation. Culturally relevant materials can be used to elicit communication, such as:

- culturally relevant books, songs, rhymes, and narratives;
- photographs from family or community functions;
- toys and objects which reflect the patient's experiences;
- dolls which reflect the patient's culture and ethnicity;
- activities and procedures within the patient's experiences (for example, making rice, steaming fish, playing bocce).

The patient can be observed interacting with people they would normally interact with, such as siblings, spouse, cousins, neighbours, and so on, providing a more realistic view of the patient's communication skills. To assess communication skills across settings and partners, informal assessment methods are ideal in beyond-clinic contexts, such as home, school, or playground. However, it is important for the speech-language pathologist to analyse the results of the informal assessment in the context of the patient's cultural and linguistic background.

RIOT approach

Cheng (1997) proposes the use of ethnographic assessment with patients from diverse cultural backgrounds. She suggests that viewing assessment data through the perspective of the target culture results in more valid and less biased information. Formal standardized testing accounts for only a small portion of this assessment approach. Rather, it advocates the collection of as much information from as many different sources and contexts as possible. The RIOT acronym stands for Review, Interview, Observe, and Test, summarizing the crucial features of this approach.

Review

Cheng suggests reviewing all relevant records, documents, and background information available, such as school records, medical records, teachers' reports, and reports from other health professionals. When accessing records, it is important to recognize that some patients might go by more than one name, and might consequently have different records corresponding to those name changes. For example, nicknames may be used, or traditional names may be spelt different ways. In more traditional indigenous Australian communities patients may temporarily change their name when someone with the same name dies, so that the dead person's spirit does not linger (Patrick, 1991). Thus, it may be useful to check if the patient has any other names, or has used any other names in the past, so that all relevant records and documents can be accessed.

Interview

It is crucial to interview as many different people as possible, such as family members, teachers, peers, other professionals, and work colleagues. The aim would be to gather as much information as possible. For example:

- the patient's communication difficulties across different contexts and with different partners;
- employment history and current responsibilities;
- premorbid communication skills;
- educational history and current abilities;
- English language exposure and experiences;
- patient/family's perception of the communication disorder and expectations about assessment and treatment;
- family structure;
- primary caregivers;
- child-rearing practices;
- what the patient/family have already done to treat the problem, if anything;
- medical and development history.

Observe

The patient should be observed in as many different contexts as possible with as many different communicative partners as possible. Different contexts may include home, clinic, school, office, and park. Communicative partners may include parents, siblings, spouse, children, teachers, peers, colleagues, and employer. Apart from observing the patient's communicative turns, it is also important to observe the routines, scripts, and cues that are used as part of those exchanges. Viewing the patient's role in the interaction as a whole will provide an insight into their linguistic as well as pragmatic abilities, such as turn taking, repair strategies, topic maintenance, and style shifting (in response to a new partner). Verbal output and comprehension should be considered, as well as language preference, bilingual competence (if applicable) and the family dynamics.

Test

Testing accounts for the smallest part of the RIOT procedure. The vast majority of information should be gathered using the other three methods.

However, testing does have a place. Cheng suggests that, where applicable, patients should be tested in both home and second languages. English-language formal assessment tools, if used, should only be used descriptively with modified scoring, and addition of culturally relevant materials. Informal assessments should make use of culturally relevant stimuli and all results should be viewed through the perspective of the patient's dominant cultural and linguistic background. Assessment should also be dynamic, evaluating the patient's ability to learn, using a test–teach–test method. Dynamic assessment is explored in more detail later in this chapter.

Issues in bilingualism

In today's multicultural and multilingual societies, knowledge and use of more than two languages is becoming commonplace. Yet, the term 'bilingualism' seems to be favoured over 'multilingualism' in the literature. Thus, 'bilingualism' is used throughout this text as incorporating 'multilingualism'.

Grosjean (1992) defines 'bilingualism' simply as 'the regular use of two (or more) languages' (p. 51). Hamers and Blanc (1989) report that definitions of 'bilingualism' vary in the literature, from the popular view of bilingualism as the ability to speak two languages with native-like proficiency to a broader perspective, which includes speakers with only minimal proficiency in their second language. However, Hamers and Blanc argue that these definitions are often problematic because they tend to lack description of what is meant by native-like proficiency or minimal competence. In addition, Hamers and Blanc argue that these definitions tend to focus on bilingualism as a unidimensional concept involving language proficiency only, ignoring the non-linguistic and cultural aspects of communication competence. Cheng (1996) suggests the need to move beyond bilingualism and towards a view of communicative competence that includes 'the individual's ability to integrate language, culture, social knowledge, and cognition' (p. 10).

Grosjean (1992) discusses two theoretical views of bilingualism — the monolingual (or fractional) view and the bilingual (or wholistic) view. According to Grosjean, a bilingual person would be defined as 'two monolinguals in one person' using the monolingual (or fractional) view of bilingualism. This view suggests that for each language a separate collective of communication proficiencies develops and that these should be directly comparable to the communication proficiencies of monolingual speakers in each corresponding language. However, Grosjean argues in favour of the bilingual (or wholistic) view of bilingualism. This view avoids comparing bilinguals with monolinguals, recognizing instead a uniquely compounded collective of language proficiencies. He uses the analogy of a high hurdler to illustrate this point (p. 55):

> The high hurdler blends two types of competencies, that of high jumping and that of sprinting. When compared individually with the sprinter or the high jumper, the hurdler meets neither level of competence, and yet when taken as a whole the hurdler is an athlete in his or her own right. No expert in track and field would ever compare a high hurdler to a sprinter or to a high jumper, even though the former blends certain characteristics of the latter two. A high hurdler is an integrated whole, a unique and specific athlete, who can attain the highest levels of world competition in the same way that the sprinter and high jumper can. In many ways, the bilingual is like the high hurdler: an integrated whole, a unique and specific speaker-hearer, and not the sum of two complete or incomplete monolinguals.

Grosjean proposes that the unique collective of communication proficiencies develops in response to the bilingual's communicative needs and experiences, so that he or she would rarely be fully competent in all aspects of each language. Rather, the bilingual's communicative proficiencies for each language will reflect his or her language use (based on topic, context, partners, and so on). Thus, Grosjean asserts that in assessing a bilingual person's communication competence consideration must be given to the 'total language repertoire as it is used in his or her everyday life' (p. 55). Just as communicative needs and experiences shape the development of language proficiencies, they also influence language loss. As communicative needs and experiences change, proficiency in one language may develop further, while it deteriorates in another. Despite this dynamic nature of language proficiency, communicative competence remains unchanged (Grosjean, 1992).

Assessment of bilingual children

Children who are bilingual follow a different path towards English-language competence compared with their monolingual counterparts. Even within the bilingual population there can be vast differences in patterns of development. In children, bilingualism can be divided into two groups based on age at exposure to the second language. Simultaneous bilingualism can be defined as the simultaneous learning of two (or more) languages, such as a child who is exposed to English and Vietnamese from birth. Sequential bilingualism implies exposure to the second language some time during or after the development of the first language (Cheng, 1991; Hamers and Blanc, 1989). Bilingual children can be expected to go through various stages of language mixing while competence in each language develops and with exposure to different patterns of language use. For example, children who speak one language at home and another at school, may develop distinct vocabularies in each language, reflecting their experiences in each situation. Language mixing can be characterized by fusion, code switching, or code mixing (Meisel, 1994). Fusion, code switching and code mixing are all characterized by the mixing of words or phrases from both languages, within or across sentences. Fusion generally occurs at an early developmental stage, and represents a fused perception of language. That is, the child has not yet developed a concept of two separate languages. Code switching represents a matured perception and knowledge of how each language can be used across different contexts, topics, and situational partners. This type of language mixing may still occur within a sentence, but now reflects pragmatic competence. Code mixing, according to Meisel, accounts for those instances of language mixing which do not seem to be rule-governed (like code-switching) but which are determined by the speaking performance (for example, a speaker uses a term from their second language in a first language context when the term cannot be retrieved from the first language at that time). Code switching and code mixing are also found in adult bilingual speech.

Children who are exposed to a second language some time during or after development of a first language, may be expected to progress to bilingual language competence faster than children who are exposed to two languages simultaneously. Basic interpersonal communicative skills (BICS) describe the surface level of conversational proficiency, whereas cognitive/academic language proficiency (CALP) describes a deeper processing and use of language for academic purposes (Cummins, 1984). Cummins proposes that the context-embedded and cognitively undemanding nature of BICS represents an early stage of language acquisition, followed by development of the context-reduced and cognitively demanding CALP. Thus, children who are exposed to a second language at a time when they are at a more mature (CALP) level of language development in their first language, will be able to apply their existing knowledge of BICS and CALP in the acquisition of the second language. Cummins reports that various research studies have found that it takes around two years for a child to develop competent surface level conversational skills (BICS) but around five to seven years to develop competent academic skills (CALP) in the second language.

Hand (1991) suggests that a child's second-language development will also depend upon factors such as amount and quality of exposure to the second language and degree of relatedness of the two languages. For example, a pre-school child who is exposed to English on a weekly trip to the local supermarket may only develop a communicative system for basic greetings, leave taking, and money exchange. In contrast, a pre-school child who is exposed to English on a daily basis through television and older siblings will have a much more developed communicative system for linguistic and non-linguistic aspects of communication. The quality of the second-language exposure is also important. A child may be exposed to English on a daily basis, but the quality of the English may be poor (for example, a parent who speaks broken English). A child may have had years of English-language exposure, but their skills may reflect those of their 'teacher'. It will also be important, then, to identify the English-language competence of the child's main communicative partners. How easily children develop their second language will also depend upon the degree of phonetic and structural similarity with the home language. For example, a child learning English and German (phonetically and structurally similar) may find it easier than a child learning English and Cantonese (phonetically and structurally different).

Assessment of bilingual aphasia

When assessing an adult bilingual patient following a cerebral event or trauma Grosjean (1989) argues the need to consider his/her bilingual language use prior to injury. Specifically, he suggests asking the following questions to describe the patient (p. 12):

*   Which languages did the patient know before injury?
*   How well did he or she know them (as a function of linguistic level, language skills, styles, etc.)?
*   What were the languages used for, with whom, for what?
*   What kind of interferences occurred in the patient's speech when in a monolingual speech mode? When speaking language A? Language B?
*   Which of these interferences were of a static nature? Which of a dynamic kind? (Grosjean defines static interferences as systematic and permanent features of one language imposed upon the other language, such as accent. Dynamic interferences, on the other hand, are described as random and accidental slips in language use.)
*   How much time did the patient spend in a monolingual as opposed to a bilingual speech mode?
*   How much mixing took place in the bilingual speech mode (if and when the patient was in that mode)?
*   What kind of mixing occurred: speech borrowing, code switching, both?
*   With whom did the patient code switch and borrow?
*   How good were the translation abilities of the patient?

Grosjean goes on to suggest that assessment following injury should reflect the patient's pre-morbid language use, creating communicative contexts that would facilitate naturalistic and representative performance in the monolingual and/or bilingual speech modes. Grosjean argues that in order to assess the patient's monolingual and bilingual speech modes successfully, his or her chosen communicative partner(s) should be truly monolingual or bilingual. In the monolingual assessment phase, it will be possible to determine whether language loss has occurred, whether there has been any change in the occurrence of interference, and whether the patient is still able to keep his or her languages separate. In the bilingual assessment phase it will be possible to determine whether the patient uses the language appropriate to the context, whether code switching and language borrowing reflect premorbid patterns (amount, type, rules for use), and whether the patient's translation abilities have been affected (Grosjean, 1989).

Disorder versus difference

Differential diagnosis is often discussed as an important goal in assessment of children from bilingual backgrounds (Anderson, 1998; Cheng, 1997; Lidz and Pena, 1996; Roseberry and Connell, 1991). Does a child present with an overall language disorder encompassing both languages, or does he or she present with language difference due to second language acquisition? Given the complex nature of bilingual language acquisition, including the potential for considerable variation in patterns of development, assessment of a child's English and home language proficiencies is unlikely to be sufficient for differential diagnosis. That is, the assumption that a child's home language proficiency would be 'normal' if the language difficulty is due to language difference rather than language disorder does not hold true when that child's home language development is also influenced by his or her bilingual language environment. Earlier in this chapter code switching was discussed as a healthy characteristic of bilingual language competence. Bilingual speakers were described as able to switch between languages based on factors such as topic of conversation, situational context, and conversational partner. Thus, it cannot be expected that a child will perform like a monolingual home-language counterpart when some functions or components of communication are second-language dominant. Anderson (1998) describes how language loss is easily mistaken for language disorder. She argues that a variety of social and environmental factors can contribute to first-language loss, such as lack of support for minority languages from the host country, small or sparse minority language communities, and mixed language use in the home rather than first language only. In addition, Anderson argues that a child's home-language model (such as a parent) may have different language patterns compared with a monolingual speaker who has not been influenced by a bilingual language community (such as a native language speaker from the parent's country of origin). Thus, children's language patterns will reflect those of their language model. Language tests, even when designed for the child's home language, may reflect expectations based on monolingual developmental patterns. It is vitally important, then, to consider the child's bilingual history and interpret test results with care.

Assessment of bilingual language proficiency can be a complicated procedure. A range of assessment options is explored below.

Standardized tests

The complexities and potential problems of using English-language standardized tests on patients from diverse cultural and linguistic backgrounds have already been explored.

Translated standardized tests

It will always be very difficult to translate assessment stimuli into another language, given the cultural and linguistic differences between English and the target language. A patient's responses cannot be compared with the test's normative information when the language of the test and language of the patient do not match (Hand, 1991; Mattes and Omark, 1991). If a translated test is used it is important to view the results descriptively and in the context of the patient's unique bilingual history. Mattes and Omark (1991) discuss several English-language tests that have been translated into Spanish, such as the Test for Auditory Comprehension of Language (Carrow, 1973), the Boehm Test of Basic Concepts (Boehm, 1971), the Receptive One-Word Picture Vocabulary Test (Gardner, 1983) and the Expressive One-Word Picture Vocabulary Test–Revised (Gardner, 1990). In their discussion, Mattes and Omark reflect on the limitations of these tests, such as the difficulty in maintaining linguistic complexity in translation, the lack of normative data from Spanish speakers, and dialectal variations reducing test validity. Readers are directed to Mattes and Omark (1991) for further details.

Standardized tests that have been normed on a population of normal bilingual children

Hand (1991) argues that patterns of bilingual language development will vary considerably across cultural and language groups, making it difficult to identify what is normal in bilingual language development. Each child's pattern of bilingual language acquisition will be influenced by his or her individual language experiences and exposures. There is also the issue of dialect differences across regions in which a specific language is spoken. Indeed Mattes and Omark (1991, p. 80) write 'The development of nationally standardized tests valid for all bilingual children . . . is unrealistic because of the heterogeneity of the various bilingual groups within this country.' However, there are numerous tools available for the assessment of languages other than English. Unfortunately, many of these reported in the literature are for Spanish only, reflecting the large Spanish-speaking population of North America and the consequent need for the development of assessment measures for this language group. Without doubt there are many more assessment tools that have been developed for other languages but have not been broadly publicized or distributed. The need for clinicians to further develop these resources is discussed in greater detail in Chapter 10. Readers are directed to Mattes and Omark (1991) for a discussion of bilingual assessment tools for articulation/phonology, language proficiency, aphasia, and hearing impairment; Cheng (1991) for a list of assessment tools available for speakers of Asian languages; and Yavas and Goldstein (1998) for a discussion of assessment tools for articulation/phonology across a range of languages. The Multilingual Aphasia Examination (MAE) (Benton, Hamsher and Sivan, 1994) and the Bilingual Aphasia Test (BAT) (Paradis, 1987) are also available for the assessment of aphasia across a range of languages. Table 5.1 provides a quick reference list of those tests identified by Mattes and Omark (1991) and Yavas and Goldstein (1998).

Interpreted language samples

Cultural and linguistic differences make it difficult for interpretation to be exact. Interpreters with limited experience or little training may find it difficult to provide a reliable interpretation, perhaps unintentionally 'filling in' for the child's linguistic errors (Isaac and Hand, 1996; Hand, 1991). The use of interpreters and the process of interpretation will be explored in much greater detail in Chapter 6.

Ethnographic assessment methods

Ethnographic assessment methods have high validity because results are viewed through the perspective of the target culture — that is, responses are analysed in terms of what would be expected given the patient's cultural and linguistic background (Cheng, 1997). Often data are gathered from a variety of sources and using a variety of methods. However, ethnographic assessment is informal and results rely heavily on the amount and accuracy of information gathered regarding the patient's history, communication diffi-culties, expected skills, and cultural and linguistic makeup.

Dynamic assessment

This type of assessment approach uses the patient's learning potential as indication of language disorder or difference via a pre-test-intervention-post-test format (Cheng, 1997; Lidz and Pena, 1996). Lidz and Pena suggest that dynamic assessment is particularly suited to children from diverse cultural and linguistic backgrounds because of the focus on how children learn rather than what they know. Mattes and Omark (1991) also discuss the importance of language learning assessment to differentially diagnose between language disorder and language difference. In examining a child's language learning potential, Mattes and Omark (1991, p. 115) suggest the following questions:

- How much structure and individual attention is required for the child to acquire new language skills?
- To what extent does the child exhibit inappropriate responses or off-task behaviours during the instructional activities?
- To what extent does the child require instructional strategies different from those used effectively with other children from a similar cultural and linguistic background?

Table 5.1. Quick reference guide to assessment tools identified by Mattes and Omark (1991) and Yavas and Goldstein (1998)

TEST TITLE	AUTHOR, YEAR
Articulation / Phonology	
+ The Austin Spanish Articulation Test	Carrow, 1974
+ La 'Meda': Medida Española de Articulación	Mason, Smith & Henshaw, 1976
+ Spanish Language Assessment Procedures (includes an articulation measure)	Mattes, 1989
+ Spanish Articulation Measures	Mattes, 1987
+ Assessment of phonological processes – Spanish	Hodson, 1984
✦ Southwestern Spanish Articulation Test	Toronto, 1977
✦ Avaliaçào Fonologica da Criança (Phonological Assessment of Child Speech – Portuguese)	Yavas, Hernandorena & Lamprecht, 1991
✦ Cantonese Segmental Phonology Test	So, 1992
Language	
+ The James Language Dominance Test (English, Spanish)	James, 1974
+ The Multicultural Vocabulary Test (English, Spanish)	Trudeau, 1985
+ Bilingual Syntax Measure (Spanish, Chinese, Tagalog)	Burt, Dulay & Hernandez-Chavez, 1978
+ Language Assessment Scales (LAS)	DeAvila & Duncan, 1983
+ Test for Auditory Comprehension of Language – Spanish	Carrow, 1973
+ Receptive One-Word Picture Vocabulary Test (Spanish)	Gardner, 1983
+ Receptive One-Word Picture Vocabulary Test: Upper Extension (Spanish)	Brownell, 1987
+ Expressive One-Word Picture Vocabulary Test: Revised (Spanish)	Gardner, 1990
+ Expressive One-Word Picture Vocabulary Test: Upper Extension (Spanish)	Gardner, 1983
+ The Screening Test of Spanish Grammar	Toronto, 1973
+ Del Rio Language Screening Test (Spanish)	Toronto, Leverman, Hanna, Rosenzweig & Maldonado, 1975
+ Pruebas de Expresión Oral y Percepción de la Lengua Española	Mares, 1980
+ Test de Vocabulario en Imagines Peabody (Spanish)	Dunn, Lugo, Padilla & Dunn, 1986

Table 5.1. (contd)

TEST TITLE	AUTHOR, YEAR
Aphasia	
✛ Examines Para Diagnosticar Impedimentos de Afasia (Spanish)	Moncada & Marshall, 1982

✛ = identified in Mattes & Omark (1991)

✦ = identified in Yavas & Goldstein (1998)

Mattes and Omark suggest that children presenting with language disorder will often require an increased need for prompts, repetition and modelling and show reduced ability to attend to the task and understand or recall information, when compared with their peers from similar cultural and linguistic backgrounds.

Lidz and Pena go on to suggest that the information gathered from dynamic assessment 'links the child's functioning to instructional strategies rather than emphasising normative comparisons' (p. 369). Thus, dynamic assessment provides an insight into the child's learning style, which will be useful for future management planning. Lidz and Pena also encourage use of the dynamic assessment model within multidisciplinary teams, thereby establishing a broad analysis of the child's learning potential across different disciplines. The pre-test-intervention-post-test nature of this assessment approach, however, requires time to complete, with monitoring of a child's performance over time. In addition, it may be necessary to consider the impact of the child's cultural background on learning style and subsequent responsiveness to the intervention phase before making judgements about the child's learning potential.

Food for thought

Given the complexities with valid and reliable assessment of bilingual language development, Hand (1991) argues that it may not even be possible to differentially diagnose a child's communication difficulty as disorder or difference. Yet, others believe that it is a crucial part of our role in assessing children from limited English proficiency backgrounds (Cheng, 1997; Lidz and Pena, 1996). Speech-language pathologists need to consider whether or not they would change their management approach if they were able to identify the cause of a child's communication difficulty as limited English proficiency due to bilingual language acquisition and not an underlying language disorder. It may be more realistic for management strategies to be based on communication competence. Competence, which can be assessed across a wide variety of settings and partners, can be used to determine functional skill. Difficulties with English-language development, due to bilingual acquisition, constitute problems with functional competence and may have a significant impact on the child's further language and academic development if left unchecked. In some clinical contexts it may be valid to establish intervention plans based on the child's functional difficulties while continually monitoring progress over time for indication of language disorder as opposed to language difference. However, when referral to special education services is in question, differential diagnosis may become a higher clinical priority. Whichever approach to differential diagnosis is taken, it is recommended that SLPs work closely with family, teachers and other professionals involved in special education and English-language programmes in order to optimize the child's language learning environment and processes.

Treatment techniques

Any intervention plans should be made with careful consideration of cultural variations (such as perceptions about the nature of the problem and expectations about treatment and outcomes), as well as linguistic variations (such as bilingual language development or the need to work with interpreters). As already suggested, functional competence may be a more realistic goal of intervention — helping the patient develop competence in the target language/s, across a variety of contexts. The SLP will need to develop his or her own cultural knowledge and competence, making use of as many resources and supports as necessary to ensure low anxiety about working with patients from diverse cultural and linguistic backgrounds. In travelling the path to cultural competence SLPs will need to critique their own cultural stereotypes, attitudes and perceptions, before cultural variation can be fully appreciated and acknowledged. Culturally focused intervention is the key and providing it requires an evaluation of everything from service delivery models to strategies for service evaluation and modification.

Service delivery

In order to provide a culturally focused SLP service it is recommended that clinics be aware of the cultural and linguistic composition of the geographical area they serve and have access to resources and information on the predominant cultural and linguistic groups, covering areas such as:

* language structure and phonology;
* religious beliefs and practices;

- attitudes towards illness and disability;
- child-rearing practices;
- family structure;
- communication/interaction styles;
- non-verbal communication;
- traditional diet and dietary habits;
- education and learning styles.

It is important to recognize, however, that for each of these areas significant intra-group variation will exist. Some families will maintain a more traditional cultural focus, while others may adopt many practices of the dominant culture. Using the information as a tool for developing ideas for and increasing awareness of alternative interpretations would be more valuable than viewing it as an inflexible dictionary of behaviours and beliefs for each cultural group. Policies and procedures for managing non-attendance and non-compliance could also be useful. Commonly used written information, such as appointment cards and handouts on language stimulation or communication strategies following stroke, could be translated into the major languages within the service's geographic area. The information contained in the handouts, however, should be culturally appropriate. A variety of service delivery models could be available for therapy, such as individual, group, school based, home based, formal, informal, sibling participation, clinician directed, or patient/parent directed.

Planning intervention

Setting goals for therapy and considering management approaches is often done in collaboration with families. When the patient/family has a different cultural background to that of the clinician intervention planning can be more challenging. Many cultural and linguistic factors need to be considered before and during planning meetings, especially if the meeting takes the form of a multidisciplinary case conference. Lynch and Hanson (1998) offer a series of guidelines for culturally sensitive intervention planning, which can be applied to both paediatric and adult clinical contexts (see Box 5.1).

It is important to remember that for any planning process the patient's/family's clinical reality should be carefully considered. This includes acknowledging their perceptions of or attitude towards the communication difficulty, their primary concerns, expectations about your professional role, and expectations about treatment (timeframe, procedure, immediacy, professionals involved, and so forth).

Box 5.1. Guidelines for culturally sensitive intervention planning

- Brief the family about the meeting, its purpose, and who will be present well in advance of the meeting.
- Reduce the number of professionals present unless the family has requested that others be present.
- Encourage families to bring those people who are important to them — relatives, spiritual leaders, friends, and so forth — and be sure that a skilled interpreter is present if families are English language learners or non-English speaking.
- Incorporate practices that are culturally comfortable for the family, such as serving tea, taking time to get acquainted before beginning the more formal aspects of the meeting, or, for some families, conducting the meeting in a highly formal manner.
- Be sure that the family input is encouraged without creating embarrassment. If it is felt that family members will not interact comfortably in such a public forum, be sure that the interventionist who knows the family best has spoken with them ahead of time and can represent their perspective at the meeting.
- Ensure that the goals, objectives, or outcomes that are being developed are matched to the family's concerns and priorities.
- Use appropriate resources that are designed for or are a part of the family's cultural community; for example, child care sponsored by the religious group to which they belong or a referral to a health-care provider who shares the same language and culture. Use cultural mediators or guides to help determine which matches are likely to be appropriate. Coming from the same country does not ensure that individuals share the same beliefs, values, behaviours or language.
- Allow time for questions, but be prepared to discuss the kinds of questions that other families often ask. This allows questions to be answered without having to be asked by family members who may feel uncomfortable about public questioning.

Source: Lynch EW, Hanson MJ (Eds) (1998) Developing Cross-cultural Competence: A Guide for Working with Young Children and their Families 2nd Ed. Baltimore: Paul H Brookes, pp. 505–6.

Intervention considerations

Lynch and Hanson (1998) suggest that 'If assessment and intervention planning are done well, the chance of conflicts arising during implementation is significantly decreased, but it may still occur' (p. 506). Thus, it is important to consider the cultural implications of chosen intervention procedures.

Therapy materials could be modified or selected to reflect the patient's experiences. This includes pictures, objects, toys, games, reinforcers/ rewards, books, songs, rhymes, computers and other technological equipment. If possible, therapy should be conducted in an environment comfortable to the patient and with the participation of people important to the patient. This type of naturalistic setting will facilitate functional intervention, low anxiety and high motivation for the patient. However, it is not always within the service's capabilities (or domain) to provide such a free-ranging approach. Hospital, clinic or school-based intervention may be the only options. In cases like this, the SLP may need to identify other methods for keeping therapy functional and motivating for the patient/family, such as inviting significant others to participate or modifying the therapy room to reflect a less formal and more comfortable atmosphere. Of course, the strategies used will depend on the patient's expectations about treatment — it may be most appropriate to use a formal setup in the therapy room, reflecting a teacher–student or doctor-patient atmosphere.

Reflecting back on bilingual language development, Cummins (1984) suggests that second-language intervention will be most successful when applied in a context-embedded situation, drawing on the child's more competent BICS (as opposed to CALP). He goes further to suggest that context-embedded learning will ultimately improve second-language skills in context-reduced situations. The implication for speech-language pathologists is obvious — create meaningful and highly contextual learning experiences to teach target goals. An example of a context-embedded intervention activity is using a multicultural calendar, as proposed by Cheng (1989b). Important holidays and events are mapped onto a calendar and used as themes for language activities, exploring vocabulary, folk tales, history, myths, and so on. The theme can be moulded to suit any language therapy goal, from vocabulary to discourse genres, and at the same time address sociocultural knowledge. Other examples include using folk tales or stories reflecting the patient's cultural experiences and encouraging the patient to bring items from home for discussion (toys, games, photos, magazines, hobby materials, food, recipes, and so on). The success of intervention will ultimately only be limited by the clinician's cultural knowledge and imagination to create relevant and motivating activities.

Which language should be used?

Where the patient is bilingual it may be confusing to decide which language therapy should be conducted in. I often hear/read of case studies where one of the SLP's main concerns is to identify which language to use in treatment. Indeed, it can be a perplexing question. It is hoped that the following guidelines help to make the decision easier. When deciding which language to use, consider the following:

In which language does the communication difficulty occur?

- Use the language the patient is having trouble with. If both languages are involved more consideration is needed.

What are the intervention goals?

- To answer this question you need to have considered your clinical goals as well as the patient/family's personal goals and expectations. The goals should reflect the patients' areas of difficulty and their functional ability (within the family domain, or, more broadly, within the community/ school/workplace). Use the language you and the patient/family have identified for that goal. If the goal involves both languages, further consideration is needed.

What degree of involvement can you expect from the family? School?

- Family and/or school support may open the opportunity to provide therapy in both languages — you focus on one, while the family/school focus on the other. This can be very effective when therapy goals encompass both languages, but can also work when goals are different.

If family involvement is available, who will be the main therapy providers?

What is the language competence of the primary home therapists? In the home language? In English?

- If home therapy is to be used, the language chosen will depend on the home therapist's competence in English and the home language. It will be important to choose the language that matches the home therapist's competence. For example, if the grandmother is identified as primary home therapist, it may be most appropriate for her to use the home language. If an older sibling is used, however, it may be acceptable to use English.

If school involvement is available, who will be the main therapy providers?

What is the language competence of the main school therapists? In the home language? In English?

- Again, it will be important to match the language with the chosen therapist's competence. Where the school therapist is competent bilingually, the chosen language should reflect each goal of therapy.

Does the SLP service have access to trained interpreters?

• Access to interpreters will open the opportunity to provide therapy in both languages in the clinical setting.

In deciding which language to use, then, it is vital to consider the therapy goals and supports. There is no reason why therapy must be provided in one language (unless the patient is only having difficulty in one language). In contrast, it will probably be more functional and salient to the patient/family to provide the opportunity to practice in both languages. Goal planning should be specific and detailed, identifying the contexts (settings and partners) and language/s each communication problem occurs in. The language identified in the goal should be the one used in therapy. Many speech and language goals will be specific to one language because of the phonetic and structural differences between the home language and English. For example, it would be pointless to work on gender pronouns in Cantonese when these do not exist in that language. Thus, therapy must be conducted in English. Goals that cross language boundaries, however, such as word-retrieval and narrative, may be targeted in both languages. It can be useful to select one language to act as the carrier language — this will be the language used by the SLP. The other language can be used at home or school, as appropriate, and intermittently reviewed by the SLP in the clinical setting. Goals that may be subject to cultural variation, such as narrative structure, should use the language matching the cultural style being addressed. Figure 5.1 shows a flow diagram for the decision on which language to use.

Evaluating and modifying

As with any service, it will be important to regularly review, evaluate, and modify intervention goals, procedures, and service policies. Be aware of cultural variability in non-verbal communication and ways of expressing dissatisfaction. Non-attendance and non-compliance may indicate a service that does not meet the patient/family's expectations or reflect their understanding of the communication disorder. It can also be useful to liaise with community leaders, for suggestions of ways to improve the overall service and make it more accessible and equitable for patients from their cultural group. Lynch and Hanson (1998) offer a range of useful suggestions for service evaluation, these are listed in Box 5.2.

Evaluation at a patient level is important, but service-level assessment and modification will ensure that clinical procedures and policies remain optimal for managing patients from culturally and linguistically diverse populations. Cultural competence has already being discussed as a key factor in maintaining a high standard of care for patients from cultural and linguistic

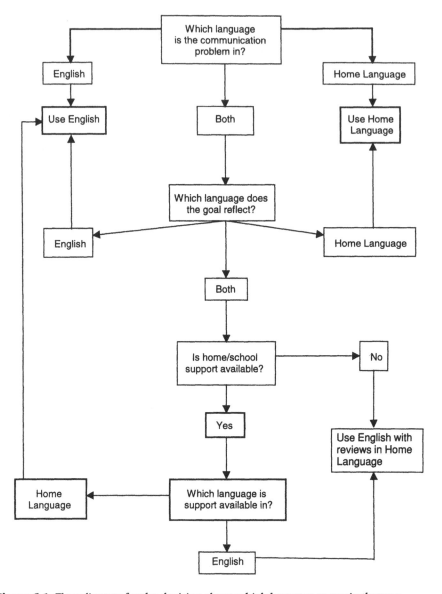

Figure 5.1. Flow diagram for the decision about which language to use in therapy.

minority groups. Ongoing education is a valuable tool for ensuring staff are up-to-date with issues relating to intercultural communication, multicultural health care, and working with interpreters. Education and research is discussed in further detail in Chapter 10.

Box 5.2. Suggestions for service evaluation

- Ensure that individual child progress or change is systematically monitored and evaluated in order to determine if goals are met within prescribed timelines and conditions.
- Develop an evaluation plan using culturally competent external evaluators to assist in the design and analysis. External evaluators have no vested interest in the programme/agency and may provide a helpful and objective examination of the practices that are effective and those that need revision.
- Develop ways to examine the degree to which families are accomplishing the outcomes that they have specified. Consider practices such as goal attainment scaling, interviews, or other unobtrusive, family-oriented approaches to gathering this information.
- Be sure that families' perceptions of the programme/agency are assessed on an annual basis. Find a system for doing this that is most appropriate for the families being served. Consider using a combination of face-to-face interviews and short questionnaires in the families' languages.
- Seek input from other community members (e.g., human services agencies, university personnel and members of cultural advocacy groups) regarding their perceptions of the programme/agency and its effectiveness.
- Maintain logs of staff development activities, new initiatives, and innovative ideas on which the programme/agency is working and revisit the program/agency's progress at least annually.

Source: Lynch EW, Hanson MJ (Eds) (1998) Developing Cross-cultural Competence: A Guide for Working with Young Children and their Families 2nd Ed. Baltimore: Paul H Brookes, p. 509.

CHAPTER 6

Different culture, different language

So far, only interactions involving shared language and different cultural backgrounds have been discussed. If shared language is also removed from the equation, so that the partners in the interaction have mutually unfamiliar language and culture, the risk of communication breakdown would increase considerably (Lynch and Hanson, 1998). In the context of unfamiliar language an interpreter is commonly used to bridge the communication gap. Even when a patient speaks some English, it is advisable to use an interpreter if there is any doubt about the patient's English-language competence. Failure to do so can have disadvantageous results for the patient.

Consider the following example in which Linda Haffner, an interpreter, recounts an experience where she interpreted for a Spanish-speaking patient who was visiting her doctor for an ante-natal check-up. On previous visits no interpreter was used, as the physician had some command of Spanish and the patient was able to speak some English. At the last visit the physician had prescribed the woman Sitz baths to aid with reducing the swelling in her hands and arms. However, during her next visit, the interpreter was called in to help determine why the patient had lost weight since last seen. As Haffner recalls:

> . . . the patient asks me to tell the physician that her hands are still hurting, but she proudly adds that she has been very good about doing her Sitz baths. She says, 'They are very tiring, but I have been doing them for 20 minutes twice a day.' I ask her to tell me what she has been doing because I wonder how a bath could be so tiring. Very seriously, she explains she would fill the tub with water and get in and sit down. Then she would stand up, sit down, stand up, sit down, stand up, sit down — for 20 minutes at a time. No wonder she was tired!
>
> (Haffner, 1992, p. 258)

As Haffner points out, this miscommunication could have had disastrous results for the pregnant woman, especially if she had fallen. This example illustrates the importance of being aware of the patient's English-language proficiency before making any recommendations without an interpreter. At the very least, it would have been valuable if the physician had described what he meant by Sitz baths, and perhaps checked the patient's understanding. However, as has already been discussed, cultural differences span across many more issues than just the issue of language. That is, even if the physician had checked whether the patient understood what he meant by Sitz baths, there would have been no guarantee that she would admit to him that she had not understood, perhaps for fear of conflicting with the physician or fear of troubling him further. In cases like this it may be better to check understanding by asking the patient to explain the procedure back. This type of checking would also avoid any instances when the patient believes they understand, but have actually misunderstood. In the example by Haffner, above, the patient may have thought she understood what the physician meant by Sitz baths because of the literal phonetic interpretation of the term Sitz ('sits'). This type of breakdown in communication could be attributed to the physician's lack of awareness of how professional jargon may not be understood by patients, or, more likely, that a patient may interpret recommendations literally. In the above example, the breakdown may be the result of a combination of literal interpretation, use of unexplained professional jargon, and an over-reliance on limited shared-language skills.

The process of interpretation

The process of interpretation has been described as 'decoding of a message in one language and its encoding in a different language' (Hamers and Blanc, 1989, p. 244), and as 'a very complex clarification and explanation of ideas from one language to another and from one individual to another' (Hatton, 1992, p. 55). These explanations seem to weigh more heavily on the role of language transmission in the process of interpreting and are similar to the code model of communication. This process could be shown as in Figure 6.1.

I have termed this process *literal interpretation* (Isaac, 2001a) because it involves only the decoding and encoding of the language component of the message being communicated. In translation, attention to the words only can result in some very humorous, if not embarrassing, statements:

- Polish tourist brochure: 'as for the tripe served you at the Hotel Monopol, you will be singing its praises to your grandchildren as you lie on your deathbed'.
- Leipzig elevator: 'do not enter the lift backwards and only when lit up'.
- In Taiwan, the translation of the Pepsi slogan 'come alive with the Pepsi generation' came out as 'Pepsi will bring your ancestors back from the dead'.

(source: unknown/anonymous)

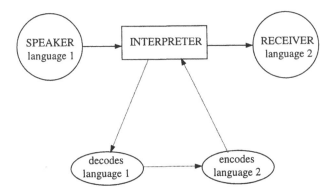

Figure 6.1. A model of literal interpretation showing language decoding and encoding only.

In verbal language interpretation, attention to the words only can have significant repercussions for the patient and/or professional:

> A foster care worker asked a youth from Vietnam if he wanted to go to school. Receiving an affirmative answer through the interpreter, the worker made extensive arrangements for the refugee to enter high school. Three months later, the youth received a straight-F report card that showed numerous absences. Further questioning determined that the youth had not wanted to go to school but had said that he did in the hopes of pleasing the worker. The interpreter was aware of this but had informed the worker of the client's statement without communicating the fact that it was not true.
>
> (Baker, 1981, p. 392)

In this example by Baker, the Vietnamese youth had agreed to going to school 'in the hopes of pleasing the worker', not because he wanted to. The behaviour of conformity to perceived authority is a cultural characteristic that has failed to be transmitted in the interaction, resulting in much time and effort spent organizing what was later found to be an inappropriate intervention.

While Hamers and Blanc (1989) state that interpretation requires that 'the content of the message is kept intact' (p. 244), in the light of the above examples, and others like it, it seems more important that the *intent* of the message is kept intact. That is, as communication is influenced by cultural factors that determine the rules for effective and appropriate communication in any situation, it follows that the interpretation process should account for such cultural influences. This process of interpretation, which I have termed *complete interpretation* (Isaac, 2001a) could be shown as in Figure 6.2.

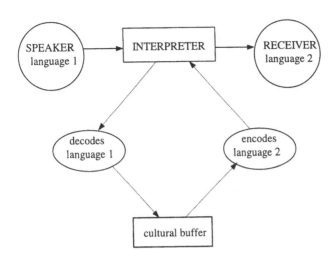

Figure 6.2. A model of complete interpretation showing the message being passed through a cultural buffer before being encoded into the target language.

The model of *complete interpretation* shows the message passing through a cultural buffer that serves to identify any cultural characteristics that may alter the intent of the message, if not considered in the interpretation. Once recognized, the interpreter can make any necessary adjustments to the message when encoded into the target language. Similarly, if the encoding does not sufficiently allow for the cultural difference to be explained, the interpreter would have the power to discuss this with the professional or client. In the situation where the professional says to or asks the client something that is potentially offensive or culturally insensitive, the cultural buffer provides an avenue for identification and rectification of this, before encoding into the target language.

Activity 6.1

If you have some experience in working with interpreters, identify and describe an episode which left you feeling that the process or outcome of the session was less than satisfactory. What was it that made you feel that way? If you do not have experience in working with interpreters, consider what you think would have to happen to make the session less than satisfactory.

In reflecting on your experiences in interpreter-mediated sessions to address this question you may have identified points similar to the following:

• your lack of experience in working with interpreters and therefore lack of understanding about their role and needs;

- the interpreter's lack of experience working in speech-language pathology or other health disciplines and therefore their lack of understanding about your role and needs;
- feelings of anxiety and uncertainty about assessing/treating a patient through an interpreter;
- little or no time for researching into relevant aspects of the patient's culture or language;
- use of an untrained interpreter whose knowledge of the patient's culture and/or language may have been less than satisfactory;
- use of an untrained interpreter whose age, gender, or social standing may have impeded rapport and perhaps professional respect for you and/or the interpreter — for example, using a younger female interpreter for an elderly man or using a younger family member and therefore disrupting the family hierarchy;
- the interpreter and patient had different cultural backgrounds despite speaking the same language;
- there was little or no time available for pre-session briefing with the interpreter;
- an interaction occurred between the interpreter and patient in which you were not involved and that left you feeling out of control of the session;
- uncertainty about how to address suspected breakdowns in communication or errors in interpreting;
- you were unable to gather the information required to make a diagnosis or plan appropriate management;
- poor time management — attempting to accomplish too much in the session.

These points are fairly general, and it is possible that you have identified additional issues specific to your own experiences. Whatever your reasons for feeling less than satisfied with your interpreter-mediated interaction, it is important to recognize that they are valid feelings but ones from which you need to learn in order to adjust your work style so that future interpreter-mediated sessions are improved. It may be useful to consider the factors influencing the interpretation process (discussed later in this chapter) to identify how your points have worked to impede the interpretation process.

Interpreter-mediated communication

A model of interpreter-mediated communication has been proposed that reflects Sperber and Wilson's (1995) inferential model of communication. As explained by the inferential model of communication, each partner within the interaction has assumptions, standards, and views of the world that are influenced by their individual experiences. In health-related interpreter-mediated communication the usual people involved in the interaction are the clinician, patient, and interpreter. Each brings his or her unique assumptions to the interaction. Since it is the interpreter who acts as a bridge between the clinician and patient, there are two separate databases of shared assumptions that develop. One develops in response to the knowledge shared between the interpreter and clinician, and the other develops in response to the knowledge shared between the interpreter and patient. It is the knowledge in these two databases that is drawn upon during the course of interpreter-mediated intercultural communication (Buchwald, Caralis, Gany, Hardt, Muecke and Putsch, 1993). Consequently, successful communication depends upon the degree to which the encoded message is understood as intended by the speaker, through the receiver finding a matching standard from their pool of assumptions. That is, the overlapping areas (databases) must be sufficiently similar.

If we are to believe that interpretation should, ideally, involve consideration of language and culture then it is not enough for an interpreter to only be bilingual. Indeed, they should also be *bicultural*. Furthermore, they should be competent bilingually and biculturally. Any person who is able to speak another language but has limited awareness and understanding of the cultural characteristics of the health professional or patient may inadequately use the cultural buffer system. Thus, a message may be interpreted in a way that reflects the cultural norms of the culture in which the interpreter is competent — reflecting narrow categorization, and possibly resulting in the transmission of false negative information. If a clinic only has ready access to family members, friends, and bilingual staff members to act as interpreters, special consideration should be given to their skills in successfully interpreting the linguistic and cultural components of the messages, so that communicative intent is accurately maintained and so that the information transmitted is culturally sensitive and appropriate to the situation. Many examples have been cited in the literature that demonstrate the potentially harmful effects of using interpreters who are not competent in one or both languages and/or cultures. Consider the following examples:

Next I am called to the Emergency Department. When I arrive, the room is full of physicians and nurses. Among them is an X-ray technician busily taking an X-ray film of a man's leg. The patient, a 38-year-old Mexican gardener, had fallen out of a 10-foot high tree. After I introduce myself, the physician and I ask the patient routine questions. The man keeps repeating, 'Mi canilla, mi canilla'. Somebody else in the room knew a little Spanish, which explains to me why the technician is taking X-rays of the man's leg. I tell them he means his wrist, which turns out to be broken. In most Spanish-speaking countries, canilla means shinbone and the use of canilla for the wrist is a little unusual — except in certain parts of Mexico where the word means wrist.

(Haffner, 1992, p. 258)

In this example by Linda Haffner, one of the health-care workers knew a limited amount of Spanish and was able to translate 'canilla' into 'shinbone'. Unfortunately, in this case, the health-care worker was not aware that the word can take on different meanings depending on the region from which the speaker comes. Health-care workers can only use the meanings they have learned and without the knowledge of linguistic variation can only continue to assume that the patient is concerned about his leg. Thus, again we see that language competence is not enough for successful interpretation. The cultural and dialectical variations of words must also be considered. This can make it difficult when arranging for an interpreter to attend a session, as some languages, such as Spanish, span across different regions as well as countries, resulting in some very different cultural characteristics. Even a trained interpreter may not be familiar with every culture in which a particular language is spoken. For that reason, then, it is ideal to identify what country or region a patient comes from before arranging an interpreter, so that one with matching culture can be found. If this is not possible it is important to be aware of the potential linguistic and cultural variations that may exist between the patient and interpreter, and to be aware that this may have an influence on the success of your interaction.

In addition to being aware of the personal culture of the patient and professional, it is also important for interpreters to have an understanding of the culture of the health profession or health-care context they are working in. This includes developing an awareness of common procedures in assessment and treatment and common terminology. Consider the following example from Putsch:

A Navajo woman was being interviewed prior to therapy with intravenous antibiotics. The nursing aide was frequently sought out by the physician staff because of her interpretation skills. She had been serving as an interpreter for 15 years.
Physician: M would you ask her if she is allergic to any medications?
Aide (in Navajo): Does the white man's medicine make you vomit?
Physician: Did you ask her if the white man's medicine makes her vomit?
Aide: Yes.
Physician: That's not quite what I need to know, I have to know about allergies to medication . . .
Aide: Well, I don't know about those things . . . what's allergy mean anyway?
If you know so much Navajo, why don't you ask her?

(Putsch, 1985, p. 3346)

In this example, a nursing aide is used as interpreter because of her perceived skills in both English and Navajo. Yet, she is not fully competent in the culture of the health profession (the culture of medicine and the meaning of *allergy*). When this occurs a number of scenarios may result:

- The interpreter may ask for clarification of the term before encoding it into the patient's language. This will allow the health professional to provide an explanation of the term or another term with which the interpreter is familiar and that he or she is able to translate accurately.
- The interpreter may not ask for clarification, feeling that he or she understands the term. This may result in the interpreter using their own understanding of the term, which may be limited or inaccurate, for example translating 'allergy' as 'make you vomit'.
- The interpreter may not ask for clarification but is aware that they are unfamiliar with the term. This may result in the interpreter guessing at the meaning, or using the English-language term in the translation.

A professional interpreter may be trained in a specific area of interpreting, such as health-care interpreting, court interpreting, or conference interpreting. If this is the case, it would be ideal to arrange an interpreter with the appropriate background knowledge. However, even an interpreter who is trained in health-care interpreting would not necessarily be familiar with all the terms and labels used in the extensive range of disciplines that fall under the health-care umbrella. Thus, as will be discussed later, it is particularly important that any discipline-specific terminology (jargon) be explained so that accurate interpretation of your message is ensured. This principle applies even more so when an untrained interpreter is used (for example, bilingual staff member, family member, or patient's friend).

Professional versus untrained interpreters

Throughout this book I will refer to professional (or trained) interpreters and untrained interpreters. I define a professional interpreter as someone who has completed a tertiary (college or university) programme in interpreting and/or has been awarded professional accreditation from an interpreting/ translating body. In Australia the National Accreditation Authority for Translators and Interpreters (NAATI) sets and monitors professional standards of practice across four accreditation levels (NAATI, 1999). Interpreters and translators may elect to seek accreditation by completing a training course recognized and approved by NAATI or by passing an exam set by NAATI. Examinations set by NAATI, at the interpreter level, cover bilingual language competence as well as social/cultural awareness and ethical issues. The four levels of accreditation provide employers with a clear understanding of interpreters' level of skill. Generally, in public health care institutions across Australia, interpreters are NAATI accredited. However, training opportunities, accreditation, and monitoring bodies will no doubt show considerable variation internationally. It is not the intention of this book to provide a description of the various training programmes available in different countries. However, it is recommended that every SLP service investigate the following questions:

- Are training programmes established for interpreters in your area?
- What do these programmes involve?
- Do interpreters receive accreditation? How? What is accreditation based on (language competence only, or does accreditation involve an assessment of cultural awareness and ethical knowledge as well)?
- Does the interpreter service you commonly use have a minimal standard of professional practice for interpreters? What is this?
- Is there a code of ethics for interpreters/translators?
- If no training or accreditation programmes are available, what is the service's procedure for selecting interpreters?

I define an untrained interpreter as someone who has not received any formal professional training or accreditation from a professional interpreting/translating body. Often untrained interpreters include family members (such as spouses, children), family friends (such as neighbours), or bilingual staff employed at the clinic/workplace. When resources are limited and patient needs are immediate it is easy to see why many clinics make use of untrained interpreters:

- they are often available when you need them;
- they cost very little, if anything at all; and
- in the case of family members or friends, there is already an established relationship with the patient.

However, the potential disadvantages far outweigh the small benefits of the above three points. As already discussed in some detail, interpreting requires not only bilingual competence but also bicultural competence, and perhaps even tricultural competence if we include the culture of the health-care context. When using untrained interpreters, language and cultural competence may not be guaranteed. In the case of family members and friends it would be difficult to determine just how competent they are in either language. It may be, for example, that the friend is a second-generation migrant who has studied and currently works in the region's dominant language and cultural environment. She may have excellent English-language skills because of this high-level and long-term exposure to English. However, she may have only a basic knowledge and ability in the patient's language and culture — enough for everyday conversation, but not enough for interpreting in a health-care context. In contrast, and probably more commonly, an untrained interpreter may have excellent knowledge and ability in the patient's language and culture but limited English-language skills. Given the many factors that are required for effective health-care interpreting, it would be unwise to use an untrained interpreter without confidence in their linguistic or cultural knowledge and ability.

Bicultural and bilingual competence are not the only predictors of effective interpreting. The chosen person may certainly possess excellent knowledge of the patient's and professional's language and culture, yet acting as an interpreter may disrupt important social and family roles. In addition, an untrained interpreter may not be bound by a code of professional ethics. This may cause some concerns regarding issues of confidentiality and impartiality. Untrained interpreters may not understand the complexities of the interpretation process, including professional roles and responsibilities, making it more difficult to establish an effective professional partnership. Lack of experience and lack of training may make it difficult for the untrained interpreter to identify breakdowns in communication and/or facilitate immediate repair.

Hornberger, Itakura, and Wilson (1997) surveyed 301 primary care physicians in northern California to determine their methods for bridging cultural and language gaps between themselves and their patients. They found that, on average, 21% of medical visits were made by patients of non-English-speaking background. The physicians also reported that in less than 6% of cases they used a professional medical interpreter. The majority of physicians chose to use untrained interpreters, such as bilingual staff members (20%) and family members or friends (36%). In 11% of cases no interpreter was used. However, physicians who had access to professionally trained medical interpreters reported a much greater perception of quality compared with untrained interpreters. Hornberger et al. also found that some physicians reported a lack of knowledge of available resources and the advantages and disadvantages of each. Woloshin, Bickell, Schwartz, Gany, and Welch (1995) also reported a lack of professional interpreter services in the public health care system in the US. They described the resulting options available to health professionals and patients as suboptimal. These options were: for the professional and patient to rely on their own (limited) language skills, to rely on family or friends, or to use untrained interpreters, such as bilingual staff or other patients. Economic restraints no doubt have a significant impact on access to professional interpreter services. Yet, it could be argued that using untrained interpreters, or no interpreter at all, would result in even greater cost (financial and otherwise) for patients, professionals, and the health-care system. Consider the following example from Linda Haffner:

The patient, a 50-year-old female peasant from Mexico, is accompanied by her 35-year-old son. Although the patient has been coming to the clinic for some time, she is new to me. Her son usually interprets, as he is reasonably fluent in both languages. This time I am called in because the son has to leave to go to work.

Before going into the room, the physician expresses to me his concern about whether the health problems claimed by this woman are real or imagined. She has been in the clinic three times before, each time with different vague and diffuse complaints, none of which make medical sense. As we learn, the poor woman has a fistula in her rectum. In her previous visits, she could not bring herself to reveal her symptoms in the presence of, and therefore to, her son as he interprets for her. She tells me that she has been so embarrassed about her condition that she has invented other symptoms to justify her visits to the physician. She confesses that she has been eager to have a hospital staff interpreter from the first visit, but her hope had not materialized until now.

(Haffner, 1992, p. 256)

Had the professional hospital interpreter been used for the first visit, this woman's condition would have been diagnosed and managed immediately. Instead, it took several visits. It could be argued that the cost in wasted time for the patient, her son, the doctor, and the health system would far outweigh the cost of employing a professional interpreter for a single visit. This example also illustrates one of the disadvantages of using family members as interpreters.

Despite the obvious dangers in using untrained interpreters, it is understood that there will inevitably be times when the needs of the patient are immediate and access to a professional interpreter is not. For example, a patient newly admitted to a hospital ward requires an urgent swallowing assessment; or during a session you realize that the patient's English-language skills are not adequate, as stated on the referral information. Perhaps the most ethical practice would be to postpone the appointment until a professional interpreter is available. When resources are limited, however, an appropriate professional interpreter may not be available for hours, or even days. This creates a significant ethical dilemma — one that clinicians need to address and solve on their own (or within their team). If the choice is made to continue using an untrained interpreter care must be taken to be highly aware of the cultural and linguistic barriers that will be present. The following chapters address more specific issues in working with interpreters, such as pre-session briefing, barriers to successful communication, and building partnerships. All the information can be applied to encounters with professional and untrained interpreters. However, it is suggested that the recommendations for improved practice carry significant weight when working with untrained interpreters.

Styles of interpreting

Interpreting can be performed consecutively or simultaneously to the speaker's message. Consecutive interpreting has been described as interpretation of the message by the interpreter after the speaker has stopped speaking. That is, each participant in the interaction takes turns, so that there is no overlapping speech (Barnett, 1989). Simultaneous interpreting is characterized by periods of overlapping speech, so that the interpreter interprets the message of the speaker as it is being spoken (Barnett, 1989; Grasska and McFarland, 1982). Each interpreting mode is designed to achieve different ends, so that consecutive interpreting may be more appropriately used in health-care encounters, such as gathering case history information from a patient, or explaining management goals; situations where the speed of message transference is not as important as establishing and maintaining patient rapport. Similarly, simultaneous interpreting may be more appropriately used in political conferences or media interviews, where the speed of message transference is paramount and the need to establish and maintain rapport less consequential, for example.

Depending upon the nature and the linguistic needs of the interaction, a message may be transferred by a number of substyles — generally, word-for-word or summary interpretation. For example, a message may be interpreted consecutively using a literal or word-for-word translation, or a summary translation. Barnett (1989) identified two forms of literal interpretation — word by word and sentence by sentence. She identified paragraph-by-paragraph interpreting as a form of summary interpreting. Several authors have identified a range of styles of interpreting related to how involved the interpreter is in the interaction. Baker (1981) proposed a model that places interpreting styles on a continuum (see Figure 6.3). At one extreme of this continuum is a style of interpreting identified as 'verbatim'. In this style, the interpreter strives for linguistic accuracy, in trying to repeat everything the clinician says word for word. Hatton and Webb (1993) used the analogy of the interpreter acting as a 'voicebox' to describe this kind of interpreting. However, in striving for a maximum degree of linguistic equivalence, the net effect is that the patient's emotions and/or cultural variations (which can have a considerable influence over the course and content of the interaction) may go unrecognized. As previously discussed, the interpreter's role is as much to culture as it is to language. Thus, 'verbatim' interpreting is likely to be inadequate in communicating the full meaning of a message.

At the opposite end of the interpreting continuum, Baker (1981) described 'independent intervention'. In this style, the interview process is controlled by the interpreter, so that they become an active participant in the

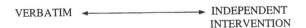

VERBATIM ◄─────────────────► INDEPENDENT
                                INTERVENTION

Figure 6.3. The interpreting style continuum, showing the extremes of verbatim interpreting and independent intervention, as described by Baker (1981).

interaction, making judgements and interjecting information without invitation from either the clinician or the patient. Hatton and Webb (1993) described this style as the interpreter acting as an 'excluder', and reported that clinicians were often left with a sense of being cast aside when the interpreter took control of the interaction with the patient. This style of interpreting becomes problematic when the interpreter assumes too much control and begins taking on responsibility and offering information that he or she may not be qualified to give. In empowering the interpreter, the clinician may be less able to guide the direction of the interaction. The clinician may begin to feel like an unnecessary presence, and the patient may lose respect for the clinician's presumed authority.

The effect of the variations in interpreting have led to recommendations about what style of interpreting is considered 'ideal'. According to Baker (1981), the ideal interpreting style lies somewhere in the middle of the continuum, borrowing a little from the characteristics of each extreme. However, he acknowledges that the exact position of the 'ideal' style will vary depending upon the nature of the interaction and the personalities of the participants. He stipulates that the interpreter and clinician must work with each other and strive to achieve a close working relationship, each contributing to the interaction the skills that are most suited. Another term that has been used to describe this ideal style is 'collaborator', indicating that the clinician and interpreter work in collaboration with each other, each one viewing the other as a colleague (Hatton and Webb, 1993). During this type of interaction, control is shared between the interpreter and clinician. Thus, interpretation is not just the responsibility of the interpreter but requires the participation of the clinician as well, the two working in partnership (see Chapter 9).

Factors influencing the interpretation process

Interpretation is a complex process, requiring that a message be transferred into a completely different linguistic code without altering the intent of the message. Interpreters should ideally have bilingual and bicultural competence so that messages can be culturally decoded. For the process of interpretation to be as successful as possible though, the interpreter and clinician must work together, in partnership. There are, however, factors that can impede the interpretation process, and other factors that enhance it. These are factors that apply to both the interpreter and the health-care professional.

The process of interpretation can be impeded by:

- assumptions about the patient, their culture and behaviours;
- assumptions or ignorance about professional roles and needs;
- ambiguous communication or negotiation; and
- acting independently without regard for how the other professional can help.

Conversely, the process can be enhanced by:

- partnership between the interpreter and clinician;
- awareness of professional roles and needs;
- clear communication and negotiation; and
- shared knowledge.

Let's return to the speech-language pathology example given earlier:

'If a child is a late talker, it is always worthwhile ruling out hearing as one of the problems.'

This statement, or variations of it, would be a fairly common comment made to parents/carers in SLP assessment sessions. As SLPs we understand that hearing difficulties may contribute to delayed language development, especially chronic hearing loss. So, we know that in the above statement the cause is hearing problems and the outcome is delayed language development. But, as discussed earlier, the structure of the statement does not clearly convey the cause or the outcome to people who are not familiar with the relationship between hearing and language development.

In an interpreter-mediated SLP session, how would the interpreter know whether hearing problems can cause delayed language development or whether delayed language development can cause hearing problems if he/she is not familiar with the relationship between the two concepts? We cannot assume that the structure of our messages will clearly convey the meaning, especially when we use complex sentence structures that may not exist in other languages (for example, if-then, tag questions). But, by working in partnership with the interpreter, sharing our knowledge by explaining concepts that may not be understood, and using clear communication, the process of interpretation, and your session outcomes, will be enhanced.

Activity 6.2

Read through the following example and discuss:

- what barriers to the interpretation process exist in this example?
- what could be done to improve the interaction? Think about the process and the roles and skills of Gabrielle and the doctor.

> Gabrielle is a foreign graduate student from a Latin American country. He has a good command of English and has very few problems communicating with his peers or following his classes. Like many graduate students, he would like to have some extra income so he decided to use his knowledge of two languages and offer his services as an interpreter . . . He had very little information about his (first) assignment. The social worker who contacted him said only that the assignment would take place at a local hospital and that the patient was a middle-aged working-class Hispanic woman. He expected the staff to help him with any questions or problems he might have and to treat him as an important element in the task to be performed by the staff. When he arrived, he informed a nurse that he was the interpreter, and she told him, in a disinterested and almost annoyed tone of voice, to take a seat and wait for the doctor handling the case. He started to feel uncomfortable. Nobody came to inform him about the case and he started feeling as though they had forgotten about him. Finally, the nurse asked him, in a dry and rough manner, to follow her. In the examining room, doctor and patient were already waiting for him.
>
> The doctor barely looked up when he came in and didn't introduce himself or the patient. He seemed to be in a hurry and apparently did not consider it important to brief him on the case. The only background information he gave was that the woman had been having abdominal cramps for a few days. When he started the interview, he spoke very fast, never looked at either the patient or the interpreter, and used technical language. Gabrielle started to feel that he was losing ground very quickly. He couldn't keep up with the speed and didn't know how or when to stop the doctor so he could start interpreting. When he finally started to interpret, he realized that he had lost quite a bit of information. By now, he was quite scared. He decided that the best way was to say what he remembered using as many similar words in Spanish as the doctor said in English, reasoning that this would at least ensure accuracy. However, looking at the patient's blank face and her responses, he realized that she was not understanding. As the interview progressed, Gabrielle grew increasingly anxious and the doctor increasingly impatient. He displayed a total lack of interest in the case, staring out the window instead of looking at the interpreter or the patient, even when the latter was pointing at the part of the body that hurt. He tried to call the doctor's attention, but was rudely dismissed implying, with an air of superiority, that he was as incompetent and uneducated as the patient.

> (Freimanis, 1994, pp. 315–16)

What barriers to the interpretation process exist in this example?

Assumptions about the patient, their culture and behaviours

- no opportunity provided for Gabrielle to familiarize himself with the patient's language register;
- no opportunity for patient, interpreter and doctor to establish rapport;
- doctor's lack of awareness of the importance of the interpreter for the patient's confidence and comfort;
- doctor's lack of eye contact with patient and disinterested tone may serve to alienate the patient.

Assumptions or ignorance about professional roles and needs

- bilingual skill is not enough to act as an interpreter — the process of interpretation is complex and requires a high level of skill in both language and cultural issues as well as knowledge and skill in professional matters such as medical interpreting, negotiation, breakdown repair, ethics, note-taking, interpreting styles, and so on;
- lack of information provided to Gabrielle regarding the needs of the doctor and what was expected of him as interpreter;
- lack of information provided to the doctor regarding Gabrielle's role and interpreting needs;
- no opportunity for rapport or the establishment of a working partnership between Gabrielle and the doctor;
- rushed feeling — poor time management;
- doctor's fast rate of speech, long sentence length, and use of professional jargon making it very difficult for accurate interpretation.

Ambiguous communication or negotiation

- no opportunity to discuss how breakdowns could be repaired;
- lack of knowledge/skill in addressing identified problems with the doctor;
- doctor's use of professional jargon without explanation placing the responsibility of accurate interpretation on Gabrielle;
- use of word-for-word interpretation is not always accurate as many terms may not be directly translatable due to lack of linguistic equivalents.

Acting independently without regard for how the other professional can help

- Gabrielle did not request clarification of jargon terms, using his own interpretation instead, which was not understood by the patient;

- doctor's lack of interest in Gabrielle's professional assistance - particularly the danger in assuming that an interpreter is merely an instrument of language interpretation and has no role in the interaction between the patient and doctor. This can result in the disregard for many non-verbal cues which can be an important part of the communication process.

What could be done to improve the interaction? Think about the process and the roles and skills of Gabrielle and the doctor.

Partnership between Gabrielle and the doctor

- time allowed for establishment of rapport, for example exchanging social courtesies;
- time allowed for discussion and therefore understanding of each other's professional role.

Awareness of professional roles and needs

- training provided to Gabrielle to better prepare him for the demands of interpreting;
- improved time management within the appointment;
- training provided to medical staff (nurse and doctor) to better prepare them for the complexity of interpreting and their roles and responsibilities (medical staff could either pursue this individually or attend an organized training session if available);
- slowed rate of speech with regular pausing to allow for interpretation.

Clear communication and negotiation

- time allowed for pre-session briefing to discuss roles and needs, procedures, expectations, and methods for breakdown repair;
- explanation of jargon terms to allow for more accurate interpretation;

Shared knowledge

- information shared regarding aims and expectations of the clinical session;
- roles and needs of both Gabrielle and the doctor discussed;
- clinical procedures discussed, including question types, preparing Gabrielle for the interpretation.

CHAPTER 7

Issues in interpreting – pre-session briefing

Meeting with the interpreter before the session is a contentious issue because the patient/parent/carer may view this as collusion between the interpreter and clinician, which may result in reduced trust and fear or anxiety about the appointment (Frey, Roberts-Smith and Bessell-Browne, 1990). However, pre-session briefings have a place in interpreter-mediated interactions and are in fact important when the session involves processes or procedures with which the interpreter is unfamiliar and therefore needs to be aware of in order to perform their professional role to the fullest; or if the session involves processes or procedures that the health professional plans to perform but that may be culturally or linguistically unfamiliar to the patient. Pre-session briefing is needed so that the interpreter and clinician can meet to discuss any issues that may impede the progress of the session and so that they can share knowledge about procedures, roles, and professional needs. If the briefing is performed openly, with the knowledge of the patient/carer, and the patient/carer understands what will be discussed and that all information will be kept confidential, the risk of perceptions of collusion should be minimized. If patients/carers are unsure about the briefing, there is no significant reason why they should not be allowed to participate in the meeting as long as there is no opportunity for either the patient/carer or clinician to be excluded from any interaction between the other two parties — all information discussed should be interpreted.

Speech-language pathology is a specialist area of work, dealing with language and communication competence. Successful interaction between the SLP and patient/carer is crucial to assessment, diagnosis, and management. Thus, briefing is important for information to be obtained and clarified allowing for any necessary modifications to be made before the session begins. Gentile, Ozolins, and Vasilakakos (1996) explore many of the difficulties interpreters face when working in the specialized field of speech-language pathology. For example, they suggest that differences in syntactic elements between languages can significantly alter the meaning of test items designed to examine those specific syntactic features, such as tense markers, gender pronouns, or plural markers. They suggest that 'interpreters require specific knowledge of the purpose of particular test items. Changes from such items, if warranted, must be made through the closest interaction between interpreter and therapist, so as to retain the purposes of the original test' (p. 128).

Pre-session briefing is suggested as an effective and efficient tool for sharing information and developing that close interaction between interpreter and SLP. Yet, I believe that pre-session briefings are not used to their full potential in most clinical contexts. In the next sections we explore pre-session briefing in more detail, comparing two approaches (Isaac, 2001b):

- one-way pre-session briefing; and
- collaborative pre-session briefing.

One-way pre-session briefing

Consider the following example of a pre-session discussion between a speech-language pathologist and interpreter, relating to an initial assessment of a three-year-old patient (it can be assumed that greeting routines have already been performed). For SLPs with an interest in adult caseloads, an assessment of an adult patient is included at the end of this chapter.

SLP: Thanks for coming in today.
INT: No problem.
SLP: The little girl that's coming in this morning, Gemma, is 3 years old. She has been referred by her mother because I think she's concerned that Gemma's not talking very much.
INT: Not talking much. Okay.
SLP: I think the mother speaks a little bit of English, but I'm not sure how good she is, so it will be best if you could interpret for her as well as anything that Gemma says.
INT: Yes, okay.
SLP: Gemma's never been seen by a speech pathologist before, so I need to ask her mother about her medical and developmental history. I also need to find out from her mother what her main concerns are, so I can get a good idea of what sort of difficulties Gemma is having.
INT: Okay.
SLP: Then, I need to try and listen to Gemma talking as much as possible, to see what she can say . . . how many words she has and whether she is putting any words into little sentences. So, if you could just interpret anything that Gemma says, that'd be great.
INT: Okay.
SLP: Does that sound alright?
INT: Yes, that's okay.

SLP: Do you have any questions about anything?
INT: No, I don't think so.
SLP: Okay, well let's go out and see if they're here yet.

In the above example the SLP provides some important information about the child and assessment processes. However, she does not provide the opportunity for the interpreter to offer information of a cultural or linguistic nature, either voluntarily or in response to specific questions. The exchange is significantly weighted towards the SLP in a position of power and control, a one-way interaction. There is no information exchanged relating to the process of interpretation or negotiation on how the two professionals will work together to achieve their goals and the best outcomes for the session. Earlier we discussed the factors which impede and enhance the interpretation process. The factors that impede were identified as

- assumptions about the patient, culture, and observed or expected behaviours;
- assumptions or ignorance about professional roles and needs;
- ambiguous communication; and
- acting independently without regard or respect for how the other professional can help.

In the example of the pre-session discussion above, it could be argued that the SLP is impeding the process of effective interpretation. She shows little awareness of how cultural and linguistic differences may influence the interaction between her and the patient/carer or influence the interpretation. She does not question the interpreter or offer an opportunity for the interpreter to discuss her roles in the interaction and her professional needs during the session. Although the SLP provides some information about the session, it is basic and does not describe the procedures that will be used to achieve the stated goals (it is the procedures used that may be subject to the most cultural and linguistic variation). Finally, the SLP has assumed a position of power and control in the pre-session briefing that can be expected to be carried over to the session, without understanding the ways in which the interpreter can assist her achieve her goals. If this interaction had occurred between a SLP and interpreter who have worked together on many previous occasions, then it can be appropriate for there to be a brief exchange primarily about the client and session goals, without repeating discussion about roles, procedures, and culture if there is nothing new to add. However, in an exchange between two professionals who are relatively unfamiliar, or when the context or procedures are new, it is important for the interaction to involve and facilitate:

- partnership;
- awareness of professional roles and needs;
- clear communication and negotiation; and
- shared knowledge.

These are the factors that will enhance the interaction.

Collaborative pre-session briefing

Consider the next example that shows the same pre-session discussion but attempts to facilitate a process of partnership through clear communication, understanding of roles, and shared knowledge:

SLP: Thanks for coming in today.

INT: No problem.

SLP: We'll be doing an assessment of a little girl this morning, but first I'd like to talk to you about what I'm planning to do in the session and to make sure that we understand each other's needs and what we need to gather during the assessment. Have you had much opportunity to be involved in an assessment session of a young child before?

INT: I was involved in one session some time ago, of a six-year-old boy. He spoke English fairly well, so I only needed to interpret for his mother and grandmother. Since then I have mainly been involved in sessions with adult patients at the hospital.

SLP: Oh, OK, so sounds like you have a fair bit of experience with working with speech pathologists, but not so much in child assessment sessions.

INT: Yes, that's right.

SLP: OK, well I'll try to explain in some detail about what we'll be doing this morning, but if you have any questions or would like me to clarify anything, please just ask. I've had a little bit of experience with working with interpreters over the last year, but we don't get that many referrals of patients needing interpreters. So any information you have about how I can best work with you to make the interpretation process easier would be much appreciated.

INT: OK, sure.

SLP: So, the little girl that's coming in this morning, Gemma, is three years old. She has been referred by her mother because she's concerned that Gemma's not talking very much.

INT: Not talking much. OK.

SLP: I think the mother speaks a little bit of English but I'm not sure how good she is. I need to ask mum quite a few questions and then later I'll need to explain to her about the sorts of difficulties Gemma is having and how we can help her, so it'll be important for her to have the best opportunity to understand what I have to say, and also the opportunity to explain her concerns to me. So, even if she does speak a little bit of English, will it be okay to still interpret?

INT: I understand that it is important for the mother to be able to understand everything you need her to know, so I will interpret what you say. If the mother says something in English, though, do you want me to repeat that?

SLP: If she says something in English, or with some English words and I find it difficult to understand what she means, I'll ask her for clarification. If she repeats it in her own language, then you could interpret that for me. Would that work all right, do you think?

INT: Yes, I think so.

SLP: OK. We'll let's start with that. I've never met the mother before, so as I said, I'm not sure how well she can speak English. Over the phone she managed fairly well to make the appointment for today, but an assessment is quite different.

INT: Yes.

SLP: Now, Gemma has never been seen by a speech pathologist before, so I need to ask her mother about her medical and developmental history. Because Gemma is only three years of age, I need to find out if there have been any medical problems that could cause her speech and language to develop slower than normal.

INT: Okay. What sort of questions would you need to ask?

SLP: I'll need to ask her about whether there were any problems during the pregnancy or birth of Gemma, whether Gemma had any feeding difficulties as a baby, when she achieved her motor milestones, like crawling and walking, and when she first started talking. I also need to ask her about Gemma's hearing. Sometimes hearing difficulties can contribute to delayed language development. So I need to find out if Gemma has ever had her hearing tested and if she has ever had any ear infections. Do you think there will be any problems with asking her mother about these things?

INT: Sometimes in this culture it can be considered rude to ask very personal questions, like about birth and pregnancy, too soon in the interview. Although this is not the case for all people, it may be good to ask the other questions first. Then, when you come to the questions about pregnancy and birth it may help to first explain why you need to ask them.

SLP: Oh, okay, that should be fine. I'll also need to find out from her mother what her main concerns are, so I can get a good idea of the sort of difficulties Gemma is having.

INT: OK.

SLP: Then I need to try and listen to Gemma talking as much as possible, to see what she can say . . . how many words she has and whether she is putting any words into little sentences. Since Gemma is so young, and does not speak any English, the best way for me to assess her language is by encouraging her to speak as much as possible in a fun, natural sort of interaction, like playing with toys or looking at books. Usually, I ask the parent to come down onto the floor and play with the child, because a lot of children will feel shy playing with a stranger. But I have read that, in Gemma's culture, it is sometimes unusual for parents and children to play and talk with each other in this way. Is that right?

INT: Yes, traditionally in this culture parents and children do not interact much. It can be unusual for parents to play like that with their children. Mostly the children play on their own or with their siblings.

SLP: Okay. So, it may not be a good idea to ask the mother to come down onto the floor and play with Gemma?

INT: Well, what you have read is very general and it may not apply to all families. Maybe Gemma's mother will feel comfortable in playing with her. But if she is not used to doing that, you may not get the type of language you want from Gemma.

SLP: Right. So, I might ask her if she would be comfortable to do it first. If it seems that she is uncomfortable about it, that's okay. And if Gemma has any brothers or sisters that come along I could involve them in the play.

INT: Yes. Since you really want to see how well Gemma can talk, making her interact with her mum when neither of them are used to doing that may not give you the language you need to assess her properly. But as I said, this is traditionally the case — perhaps Gemma's mother may be quite comfortable playing with her.

SLP: Okay. So, when we are playing with Gemma, I need to know whether she is able to understand language, like follow directions, and how well she is able to talk. To see how well she can understand, I'll need to ask her different types of questions and directions, like 'where's the book?' 'where's the cup?' and longer ones like 'put the spoon on the plate' and 'put the doll in the car', that sort of thing. It'll be important for me to know whether she is able to understand these directions, or whether she has any trouble, like needing the question to be repeated before she does it. Do you think that would be OK?

INT: Yes, I think so. You understand that the structure of the two languages is very different and the word order may need to be changed to suit Gemma's language.

SLP: Yes. If I ask a question, then, that is difficult to interpret, would you be able to let me know? That way I can try to give you another question that will be easier and still let me check her understanding.

INT: OK. So, you want to know if any of the questions have to be repeated before she answers them?

SLP: Yes, if that's possible.

INT: OK.

SLP: It would also be great if you could interpret anything that Gemma says. I'm not sure exactly what her difficulties are and it may be that she has some trouble pronouncing the words clearly. So, if you hear her say any words that are not pronounced properly, could you let me know?

INT: Sure.

SLP: If Gemma uses any sentences, I won't know whether they are good sentences because I am not familiar with the structure of your language, so if you are comfortable to do this, it would help me if you could tell me whether her sentences make sense and use all the right bits of grammar, or whether she leaves anything out.

INT: I don't feel that I have the skill to make a judgement about her speech. I am not trained in this area.

SLP: Oh, I understand that, and I don't want to put you in a position where you feel uncomfortable. I don't want you to make a judgement about whether Gemma's language is right for her age or not, instead it would help me if you just sort of described it to me. So, tell me if she leaves something out, like the little word 'is', or if she uses a different word to name something, like 'woof' for 'dog', that sort of thing. More of a description than anything else.

INT: Oh. OK. That should be all right — as long as I don't have to tell you whether it is right or wrong.

SLP: No, no, not at all. Just a description. If I can get all the information I need, I'll spend some time at the end of the session talking with Gemma's mother to let her know what we can offer Gemma to help develop her speech or language more.

This is assuming there is a problem. If there is a problem with Gemma's speech or language then I'll need to explain to her mother what we can offer in terms of treatment. We have a fairly long waiting list for treatment though, so her mum might be happy to work with Gemma at home on a programme that I give her, while she is waiting.

INT: Yes. But, if her mother is not used to interacting with Gemma in that way, she may not be comfortable doing that.

SLP: Oh yeah, okay. If we find that to be the case, I'll see who mum suggests — perhaps a pre-school programme would work best. Okay, well is there anything else you'd like to know or anything else you think I need to know before we start?

INT: No, I don't think so.

SLP: Okay. What if something happens during the session, like I ask a question that you think may potentially offend or embarrass Gemma's mother. How should we deal with that? I think I'd like to know so I have the chance to change my question, or whatever.

INT: Yes. That would be okay. I can let you know before I interpret it, if you'd like.

SLP: Yeah, that would be great. Thanks. Well, let's go out and see if they are here yet.

This revised pre-session discussion is obviously longer than the first one and involves much more collaboration and sharing of knowledge. It meets the criteria for facilitating a partnership between the professionals by demonstrating an awareness of professional roles and skills and how they can be used in the session, clearly communicating and negotiating processes and procedures, and demonstrating an awareness of the cultural and linguistic variations between the SLP and patient/carer. The SLP, although still providing and requesting the majority of information during this exchange, provides the opportunity for the interpreter to offer information and discuss issues that may influence the interaction between the SLP and patient/carer or influence the outcomes of the session. The two professionals are working together to establish processes and procedures which will result in the best outcomes for the session.

This second pre-session briefing takes about 10 minutes to complete. It is a lengthy discussion, but achieves far more for the session than the first example would have. It is also important to bear in mind that if the SLP and interpreter had had prior experience working with each other or in similar contexts, then it may not be necessary to discuss everything that is included or to discuss it in such detail (this is why it is useful to check the interpreter's experience and to be aware of your own experiences and limitations). Pre-session briefings will vary considerably, depending upon the experience of the professionals involved and the complexity of the case. Good time management is a necessary skill — planning for the interpreter to arrive 10 or 15 minutes prior to the session will allow the opportunity for this valuable discussion. Below is a comprehensive list of the type of information that may be useful to collect and discuss with an interpreter during a pre-session briefing.

Points of discussion and negotiation

- Your experience working with interpreters.
- The interpreter's experience working in the field of speech-language pathology.
- The interpreter's experience working in this setting and with this patient type.
- Plan of action for the session, including planned procedures and materials to be used — many interpreters may prefer to see written materials early on so that they have time to prepare appropriate interpretation or translation. If the written materials are extensive it may be worthwhile providing the interpreter with a copy some days before the scheduled appointment. Not all interpreters will feel comfortable to translate written materials. It may be necessary to obtain translations of frequently used materials through specialist translating services, if available.
- Session goals — what you hope to achieve in the session.
- What involvement you hope the interpreter to have in the session — discussion of roles.
- How the interpreter perceives his/her role in the session.
- Style of interpreting — simultaneous or consecutive.
- Interpreter's use of note taking.
- Interpreting needs — for example, rate of speech, when to pause, how to signal breakdown, and so forth.
- Methods for repairing breakdown.
- Cultural and linguistic influences on session procedures, including materials to be used, questions/language stimuli, seating arrangements, non-verbal signs, and so forth.
- Patient's/carer's background — including any information on education, employment, country/region of origin, as well as background information on the patient's communication difficulty and (if relevant) medical history. Having a brief understanding of the patient's/carer's education and employment history can help the interpreter determine the best language style to use, so that the patient is not alienated by a register that is too formal or too casual. If this information is not available or appropriate to pass on to the interpreter, it may be useful to allow the interpreter a couple of minutes at the beginning of the session to casually chat with the patient/carer to establish an appropriate communication register.
- Preparing the interpreter for unfamiliar physical presentations (for example tracheotomized patient, changing laryngectomy prostheses, cranio-facial abnormalities, and so forth) or significant behavioural issues.

Food for thought

Identify and reflect on your own experiences in pre-session briefings. How do they compare with the suggested points of discussion? Can they be improved? If so, how? Role play a pre-session briefing with a colleague, using a context that is relevant to your own workplace. Try one that assumes the interpreter has little experience working in that setting or with that patient type, and then re-do that pre-session discussion assuming that the interpreter has worked with you before on several similar cases.

If you have the opportunity to videotape a pre-session discussion with an interpreter, do so, and evaluate your performance in terms of the above points.

Pre-session briefing — adult case example

One-way pre-session briefing

SLP: Okay . . . well, the gentleman we're going to see in a moment is 73 years old and has been in hospital for a day now.

INT: Mmm.

SLP: The doctors believe he has had a stroke and have referred him to me to assess his communication.

INT: Right.

SLP: I went to see him yesterday afternoon when he first came up to the ward. He had some of his family with him, I think his son and daughter-in-law, and another lady that I think was his sister. His son could speak English fairly well and was able to give me a little information about Mr Chang's speech.

INT: Mm-hmm.

SLP: His son said that he had not spoken very much since he was admitted yesterday and seemed very drowsy. I wasn't able to find out whether what he was saying was okay or whether it sounded a bit slurred, or whether he was having trouble putting words and sentences together.

INT: Okay.

SLP: According to his son, Mr Chang speaks very little English, so I need you to help me assess his communication.

INT: How would you like me to do that?

SLP: Well, I'll need to ask him different types of questions to determine whether he has any trouble understanding what other people say to him. I also need to listen to what he can say . . . see whether he can name things, and maybe talk about a picture, to see what his sentences are like.

INT: Mm-hmm.

SLP: I need to know whether what he says sounds slurred and unclear, or whether he sounds normal but has trouble finding the right words or putting sentences together. Will that be okay?

INT: Yes, I think so.

SLP: Okay, I think that's about it. Do you have any questions?

INT: So, you need to assess his communication to see whether he has any trouble understanding or using sentences, and you'd like me to let you know if his words sound unclear. Is that right?

SLP: Yes, that's it.

INT: Okay.

SLP: All right then, I'll just grab my things and we'll go down to see him.

Collaborative pre-session briefing

SLP: Okay . . . well, the gentleman we're going to see in a moment is 73 years old and has been in hospital for a day now.

INT: Mmm.

SLP: The doctors believe he has had a stroke and have referred him to me to assess his communication.

INT: Right.

SLP: I went to see him yesterday afternoon when he first came up to the ward. He had some of his family with him, I think his son and daughter-in-law, and another lady that I think was his sister. His son could speak English fairly well and was able to give me a little information about Mr Chang's speech.

INT: Mm-hmm.

SLP: His son said that he had not spoken very much since he was admitted yesterday and seemed very drowsy. I wasn't able to find out whether what he was saying was okay or whether it sounded a bit slurred, or whether he was having trouble putting words and sentences together.

INT: Okay.

SLP: According to his son, Mr Chang speaks very little English, so I need you to help me assess his communication.

INT: How would you like me to do that?

SLP: Well, we don't know yet what type of stroke Mr Chang has had, so I can't really predict what sort of difficulties he might have — we really need to be on the lookout for anything.

INT: What sort of things?

SLP: Well, when somebody has a stroke, their ability to communicate can be affected in a variety of ways. He may be having trouble making the sounds to produce the words, or he could be having trouble finding the words he wants to say, or putting the right words into sentences. It could also mean that he has trouble understanding what other people say to him.

INT: So, you need to know about all of these things?

SLP: Yes, I'll need to know things like, whether he is saying the words clearly, or whether they are coming out slurred or mispronounced; and whether he uses any words that do not fit right or make sense in his sentence. Would it be possible to get all this information?

INT: So, when he is talking you want to know whether it sounds clear, whether he uses any wrong words, and whether he makes sense?

SLP: Yes. Will that be possible?

INT: Do you want me to interpret what he says or just tell you this information?

SLP: Well, if you can interpret what he says that would be wonderful. Sometimes though, strokes can cause people to say words that don't fit into their sentences or words that don't make any sense, and if he is doing either of these it may be hard for you to interpret. In this case, your description of what seems to be the problem would be best.

INT: Okay. So, I will interpret what he says, but if he says anything that doesn't make sense or if he sounds slurred, I'll let you know. What about his understanding? You mentioned that that can sometimes be affected by stroke.

SLP: Yes. I think I should be able to get a fair idea of his understanding from the way he responds to my questions. But, if you find that he needs you to repeat the question or change the wording of the question to make it easier, could you also let me know that?

INT: What sort of questions will you be asking Mr Chang? Because when I interpret them into his language the wording may change anyway.

SLP: Right. I'll start by just listening to how he responds to questions as part of a general conversation. I might ask him about his family, where he lives, that sort of thing. Then I might need to have a more specific look at his understanding by having him follow directions like pointing to objects I name or moving them about.

INT: The conversation questions should not be a problem. However, the directions may change slightly when they are interpreted into Mr Chang's language. If it would help I can let you know how the question would change before I interpret it, so you can determine whether it still achieves what you want. Would that help?

SLP: Yes, that would be great. Thanks. Is there anything else you think I need to know before we start, or anything else you need to know about the assessment?

INT: Something to keep in mind is that, traditionally, in Mr Chang's culture, younger females are usually not as highly regarded as men in the same position and this may have an effect on how Mr Chang interacts with you, what he says, and how he responds to your questions, especially if he does not understand why you are getting him to do all these things.

SLP: Oh, Okay. Thank you for that. I'll try to help him understand as much as possible. If it is having an impact on the assessment, though, perhaps tomorrow, if you are able to come back in, we could discuss some ways to manage that. Is there anything else?

INT: No, I don't think so.

SLP: Okay, I'll just grab my things and we'll go down to see him.

CHAPTER 8

Issues in interpreting — potential barriers

As previously discussed, miscommunication does happen between individuals who speak the same language and share the same cultural history (Buchwald et al., 1993; Lynch, 1998). However the lack of a common language and cultural background increases the amount and type of communicative difficulties that can occur. Barriers to effective and accurate communication in interpreter-mediated interactions can be divided into two categories — linguistic and non-linguistic difficulties. Since the process of interpretation involves collaboration, the success of the interaction may be influenced by the interpreter and SLP (Isaac and Hand, 1996; Hatton and Webb, 1993; Faust and Drickey, 1986; Baker, 1981).

Linguistic difficulties in interpreting

Linguistic barriers to communication are those that arise out of language-based differences. That is, miscommunications that result from:

- the lack of a common language between the clinician and patient;
- differences in word meaning between languages;
- differences in explaining culture-specific behaviours or technical information to do with assessment or intervention issues; or
- miscommunication resulting from literal or word-for-word interpretation of a message.

Paraphrasing

Several studies have reported breakdowns during the act of paraphrasing (Buchwald et al., 1993; Vasquez and Javier, 1991; Putsch, 1985; Miller and Abudarham, 1984; Diaz-Duque, 1982; Grashka and McFarland, 1982; Launer, 1978). Paraphrasing is the act of relating the speaker's message either word-for-word or in summary. Difficulties can occur when the message is only loosely interpreted so that the resulting message is somewhat different to the original. Launer (1978) performed back-translations on the interactions between interpreters, doctors, and patients in a Nigerian hospital. That is, he audiotaped interpreter-mediated interactions between doctors and patients and replayed those to a second interpreter, the aim being to investigate if any alterations were made to the original message. Launer found that some messages were indeed altered during the interpretation. He classified these errors in paraphrasing as errors that either distorted the intended meaning of the message (described as 'illegitimate deviations') or those that retained the intended meaning of the message (described as 'legitimate deviations') (Launer, 1978, pp. 934–5).

Errors that result in a loss of meaning include:

- condensation of the message, so that important information is omitted or downplayed;
- addition of information not included in the original message; and
- substitution of concepts expressed in the original message using the interpreter's own understanding of the meaning (Vasquez and Javier, 1991).

Consider the following example from Launer's study, in which the interpreter has condensed the patient's message, omitting important information and reducing the severity of the patient's symptoms.

> Patient: It's my ear that's hurting me. It's blocked and I can't hear with it. The head and the neck are hurting and I've got a fever.
> Interpreter: She says she is suffering from ear pain and headache.
> (Launer, 1978, p. 935)

Paraphrasing is often a necessary step in interpreting between two languages that have different semantic and syntactic structures, as well as cultural variability. Word-for-word interpretation would rarely result in an accurate transference of the message, especially if the message is long and complex. How accurately the intended meaning of a message is interpreted may depend upon the interpreter's understanding and/or assumptions about what is relevant for you to know, based on their understandings and/or assumptions about your aims and goals. Thus, for the interpretation to be as close to your needs as possible, the interpreter should have a clear understanding of your goals and intended outcomes. Clear communication and shared knowledge are needed to make the interpretation work to everyone's benefit.

Professional jargon

It is easy to become casual with the terms and concepts that apply specifically to your profession when you are exposed to them on a frequent basis. However, it is important to avoid the trap of assuming that patients and other professionals will understand what they mean, no matter how simple a term may seemingly be. A number of authors have advised that the use of professional jargon may lead to miscommunication during interpretation (Buchwald et al., 1993; Putsch, 1985; Diaz-Duque, 1982). If health professionals provide explanations that include discipline-specific terminology, with which interpreters may be unfamiliar, two possible scenarios can arise. Firstly, the interpreter may request clarification from the health professional and thus elicit an alternative explanation that is easier to interpret. Secondly, the interpreter may not request clarification from the health professional, going ahead with the interpretation as best they can. In doing this, the interpreter may not be able to provide a linguistic equivalent for the term and, therefore, may use the English word in the translation. On the other hand, the interpreter may attempt to define the term to the patient using their own understanding. The danger in doing this, however, is that the interpreter may not have sufficient knowledge of the clinical and/or theoretical procedures of the health profession to be able to define the term effectively and accurately, as in the example by Putsch (1985, p. 3346) discussed in Chapter 6, in which the nursing aide used the word 'vomit' to describe 'allergy'. In this example, the aide, who had been serving as an interpreter for fifteen years, did not understand the term *allergy*, and could not, therefore, provide a suitable linguistic equivalent in the translation. Instead of requesting further explanation from the physician, she attempted to interpret the message as she understood it. Putsch (1985) suggests that such discipline-specific terminology may be variably understood by individuals of the same linguistic and cultural background to the health professional, often requiring explanation. Thus, the health professional needs to be aware that 'jargon' terms may not be understood by the interpreter or translate into another language as desired.

Lack of linguistic equivalents

The repertoire of terms and concepts is different in every country. Words that are commonly used in one language, such as English, may have no equivalent meaning in another language, such as Mandarin or Russian, for example. This is especially true when terms apply to culture-specific practices, such as health practices, considering that many cultures have vastly different methods of assessing and treating illness. Consequently, lack of recognition of this fact will amplify the risk of miscommunication

(Buchwald et al., 1993; Meyers, 1992; Putsch, 1985; Grasska and McFarland, 1982).

Where no linguistic equivalent exists, the interpreter may choose to request clarification or attempt to interpret the term using their own understanding, as described in the previous section on professional jargon. Thus, it is important that the clinician and interpreter negotiate a method for repairing and clarifying potential areas of communication breakdown, prior to the session starting.

Sentence length

The health professional or patient may be unaware of how to work with an interpreter. Either one, or both, may speak too fast and in sentences that are too long for the interpreter to remember, or translate as accurately as possible (Buchwald et al., 1993; Vasquez and Javier, 1991; Faust and Drickey, 1986; Grasska and McFarland, 1982). Therefore, the risk of miscommunication becomes greater because there is a greater chance that the interpreter will not remember all the required information or that the patient will become overloaded with information that they may not understand. In an interview with Shotsy Faust and Robert Drickey one interpreter stated that:

> It takes extra time to convey thoughts cross-culturally as well as bilingually. In an effort to include all that is necessary, the provider often tries to include too much in a sentence, or there isn't time to explain all that the provider says. The patient often leaves overloaded with information and with too many things to remember to do.
>
> (Faust and Drickey, 1986, p. 137)

Some interpreters may request you pause if they feel the message is becoming too long. Others may use note-taking to aid their memory of the points discussed. Interpreting is a two-way street, clear and successful communication is the responsibility of both parties. The clinician should pause regularly, at contextually appropriate points; the interpreter should be encouraged to use note-taking if the message is expected to be longer or more complicated than normal; and strategies for repair should be discussed prior to the session so that any difficulties due to sentence length or complexity can be efficiently and appropriately addressed.

Variations in dialect or word meaning

Some languages are shared across different countries, and although the basics of the language remain the same, certain individual words may change over time, so that one word assumes a number of different meanings, which can be quite different from one another. Poss and Rangel

(1995) suggest examples of word-meaning differences across countries where the same language is spoken. For example, in the Spanish-speaking countries of Puerto Rico and Mexico *guagua* means 'bus', but it means 'baby' in Chile (p. 44).

In addition, some countries have more than one language in active use and they may be mutually unintelligible. For example, in China there is a vast number of languages and dialects spoken in different areas, such as Mandarin, Cantonese, Min, Hakka, and Toishanese (Cheng, 1993; Chan, 1992; Lee, 1989). The success of the interpreting will ultimately depend upon the interpreter's ability to understand the dialect of the patient (Dentino, 1991).

When booking an interpreter for a session, it is important to provide as much information as possible about the language which the patient speaks. Only providing a country or nationality (for example, Chinese) may not be enough and could result in an interpreter who comes from the same country but does not speak the patient's language or dialect. Similarly, as some languages span across different countries, it is important to try to book an interpreter who not only speaks the same language or dialect as the patient, but who also shares a similar cultural background.

Register

The term 'register' refers to the way language is used in particular social contexts, for example different registers may have different levels of language formality. Often, the registers we feel comfortable in reflect our educational and social background. If possible, an interpreter should be able to recognize the patient's register and subsequently alter their own language register to match. If this is not done, the patient may be inadvertently alienated from the language of the interaction, if it is at too high a register, and they may choose to adopt a more passive role in the interaction, particularly if they do not understand the questions or issues being asked or discussed. Similarly, a patient who uses a higher or more formal register than the interpreter may have reservations about the professional abilities of the interpreter and/or health professional, and may not provide all the information they otherwise would have (Poss and Rangel, 1995).

Providing the interpreter with relevant background information about the patient/carer (for example, educational and employment history) may allow them to choose a more appropriate language register. If it is not possible to provide this information prior to the session (for example, in the pre-session discussion) it may help to allow the interpreter a couple of minutes at the start of the session to casually chat with the patient/carer to determine the appropriate language register to use.

Polishing

Diaz-Duque (1982) identified polishing as another barrier to successful communication with patients from non-English speaking backgrounds. Polishing occurs when the message is rephrased using more technical language so that there is a loss of insight into the patient's emotions, which may be very instrumental in assisting the clinician to make appropriate decisions regarding current and future management issues. This example comes from Putsch:

> Interpreter to patient: Is there anything that bothers you?
> Patient: I know . . . I know that God is with me. I'm not afraid, they cannot get me (pause). I'm wearing these new pants and I feel protected. I feel good, I don't get headaches anymore.
> Interpreter to clinician: He says that he is not afraid, he feels good, he doesn't have headaches anymore.
>
> (Putsch, 1985, p. 3347)

In this example, the patient's message has been polished so that his mental health disorder has been normalized. Thus, the clinician is not made aware of the patient's true perception of their problem or their state of mind. With specific reference to SLP, polishing may include the upgrading of expressive language skills, particularly grammatical skills in children, or the language of aphasia in adults. During assessment, a speech-language pathologist aims to gather information about a patient's communication skills that allows for appropriate management decisions to be made. However, if the patient's communicative attempts are altered through the process of polishing, the SLP may (unknowingly) base decisions on inaccurate information.

Again the need to share information about your needs from the interpretation to appropriately assess the patient is paramount, as is sharing information about what the interpreter may expect the patient's language to be like, or what particular language characteristics they should look out for.

Non-linguistic difficulties in interpreting

Barriers to successful communication are not solely grounded in language. Indeed, there are numerous barriers that may arise from cultural and personal differences between the interpreter, patient, and clinician. As previously discussed, Sperber and Wilson (1995) proposed an inferential model of communication which describes the way in which miscommunication can occur between people who speak the same language and share the same cultural background (refer to Figure 1.2). Buchwald et al. (1993) use a similar model to describe why miscommunication occurs in interpreter-mediated interactions. Both these models are based on the notion that, in addition to attitudes and perceptions held common with other members of the society, every individual has other unique attitudes and perceptions. It is this discrepancy in views (based on cultural or personal differences) that may cause miscommunication to occur. Several authors have identified specific areas of such non-linguistic difficulties. These are discussed below.

Dissociation

Putsch (1985) and Grasska and McFarland (1982) suggest that a message can lose some or all of its emotional and non-verbal information during the process of interpretation, especially if there is too much emphasis placed on language interpretation. Extreme emotions may be obvious, but cultural behaviours may mask these. It is generally believed that verbal communication only carries a small amount of emotional information, whereas non-verbal behaviours convey a much greater amount of emotional information. When interacting across cultures the clinician may lose their ability to assess a patient's emotional state, since emotional signs and expression will inevitably vary across cultures. The following example demonstrates a successful interpreter–clinician interaction, in which the interpreter suggests an unusual behaviour that the clinician did not identify:

> during a visit with the Garcia family, the nurse found nothing amiss and enjoyed Ms. Garcia's good humour. In fact, as the nurse and interpreter left the Garcia residence, the nurse remarked, 'Isn't Ms. Garcia a cheerful person?' The interpreter replied, 'Yes, but she laughed at all the wrong things.'
>
> (Grasska and McFarland, 1982, p. 1377)

This is a good example of successful communication of a non-verbal behaviour that prompted the clinician to investigate the patient's mental health history. However, this information may have been overlooked or ignored if the nurse had not remarked on Ms Garcia's apparent cheerfulness. Again, this illustrates the importance of sharing information about your needs and what language and/or non-verbal behaviours the interpreter should look out for.

Independent intervention

Independent intervention is a style of interpreting described by Baker (1981) in which the interpreter assumes control over the interaction, making judgements and asking questions without direction from the clinician or patient. Hatton and Webb (1993) identified this style of interpreting between the interpreter and patient as having the effect of excluding the clinician from the interaction. Independent intervention can be shown diagramatically as in Figure 8.1.

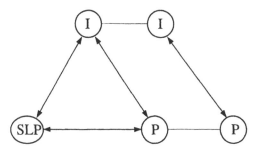

Figure 8.1. A model of independent intervention, showing the interaction between the interpreter and patient that occurs at the exclusion of the SLP.

Buchwald et al. (1993) recognized that, in any interview, the interpreter holds considerable power as both a 'channel of information and a broker of cultures' (p. 143). Despite the fact that professional interpreters are trained to remain neutral in an interaction, they can have an influence on what sort of information is presented. That is, the interpreter draws on their perception of the patient's and clinician's cultural, social, and professional background to make judgements about health care and information needs (Kaufert and Putsch, 1997; Buchwald et al., 1993; Putsch, 1985). For example:

> Acting out of concern and hoping to preserve harmony, an interpreter told a client not to tell the social worker about her problems or the anger she was feeling because the social worker 'has had a hard week and does not need any more problems to worry about'.
>
> (Baker, 1981, p. 393)

Miller and Abudarham (1984) related an experience with an interpreter during a speech-language pathology assessment session of a young child. The child's receptive language skills were being examined and the interpreter was requested to ask the questions on the question sheet exactly as they were written. The session was video recorded and later analysed by the clinician and interpreter. At one point in the testing format, the interpreter seemed to take an exceptionally long time to ask one of the questions — 'point to the bath'. Discussion revealed that when the child did not respond correctly the first time, the interpreter rephrased the question and asked the child to point to 'the thing next to the chair'. The interpreter's reason for doing this was that he believed that the child knew what 'bath' meant, and was therefore only trying to elicit a correct response. Thus, the interpreter took over control of the assessment task by changing the questioning format based on his personal judgement of what the child knew and did not know.

At times interpreters may independently intervene when they have some specialist knowledge of the clincian's profession or the particular issue being discussed or examined. Consider this next example from Kaufert and Putsch:

> Doctor: She's anemic and pale, which means she must be losing blood.
> Interpreter (in Cree): This is what he says about you. You are pale, you have no blood.
> Doctor: Has she had any bleeding from the bowel when she's had a bowel movement?
> Interpreter (in Cree): When you have a bowel movement, do you notice any blood?
> Patient (in Cree): I'm not sure.
> Interpreter (in Cree): Is your stool ever black or very light? What does it look like?
> Patient (in Cree): Sometimes dark.
>
> (Kaufert and Putsch, 1997, p. 78)

In this example, the interpreter has used her own knowledge of gastrointestinal history taking to question the patient about stool colour, to further determine whether there may be any evidence of blood. However, it is always ideal that any information exchanged at the exclusion of either the clinician or patient be interpreted back to the excluded party (Kaufert and Putsch, 1997). In this way, independent intervention at the exclusion of the clinician, as in the above examples, may be checked for linguistic and clinical accuracy.

Putsch provided an example of an interpreter who completely changed the message of the provider, in this case a psychiatrist because she believed that the psychiatrist's initiative to include the patient in the decision-making process would be seen by the patient as therapeutic incompetence:

> Psychiatrist: Ask her how long she thinks she'll need to take these medications.
> Interpreter: He says you should take this medication for two weeks and then come back to see him.
> (The return date and appointment were discussed in Vietnamese.)
> Interpreter: She says she'll take the medicine for two weeks and then she'll come back to see you.
>
> (Putsch, 1985, p. 3347)

Cultural differences between the clinician and patient, as in the example above, can also result in miscommunication or, even worse, perceptions of professional incompetence. Here, the interpreter has recognized the potential problem in the clinician's request and has altered the message to present it in a more culturally appropriate way. The situation could have been avoided had the clinician developed an awareness of the potential differences in perceptions of the role of the clinician and patient in decision making. By being aware of the potential for differences to exist across cultures in attitude towards and expectations of common professional practices (for example, history taking, questioning, decision making, physical examination, and so forth) the clinician will be better prepared to gather information from the interpreter prior to the session and negotiate avenues for repair, should the clinician say or do something that is culturally inappropriate.

Culture differences

Although individuals may be bilingual, it does not necessarily mean that they will be bicultural (Buchwald et al., 1993). This is especially the case if the country from which the patient comes is large and culturally diverse. Some languages span across different countries altogether, making it almost impossible for an interpreter to have a thorough understanding of the cultural issues pertaining to every area where the language is spoken. For example, Spanish is the official language of Mexico (North America), Honduras (Central America), Argentina (South America), Cuba (West Indies), and Equatorial Guinea (Central Africa); Portuguese is the official language of Angola (South Africa), Brazil (South America), Guinea-Bissau (West Africa) and Portugal (South West Europe); French is the official language of Niger (West Africa), Rwanda (Central Africa), Canada (North America), Haiti (West Indies), Monaco (Southeast Europe), Belgium (North West Europe) and France (Western Europe); Arabic is the official language of Sudan (East Africa), Egypt (North Africa), and Lebanon (South West Asia). Thus, an interpreter who is able to speak the patient's language but has limited knowledge of his or her cultural beliefs, attitudes, and practices may not be able to interpret information in a culturally appropriate manner. Therefore, miscommunication may arise as a result of poor cultural knowledge. This again highlights the importance of having a clear understanding of the patient's linguistic and cultural background before booking an interpreter. As illustrated above, simply booking a Spanish-speaking interpreter, for example, may not guarantee matched culture.

The melting pot

The melting pot phenomenon is characterized by the belief that minority cultures can be expected to assume the beliefs and customs of the dominant culture (Wells, 1995; Battle, 1993). That is, the clinician may assume that the patient shares his/her own views on health care, child-rearing practices, dietary habits, and so on. Indeed, some patients from non-English speaking background can be sufficiently acculturated for this to be true. However, it cannot be assumed that all patients will be fully acculturated, and therefore it is important for clinicians to be aware of cultural differences so that assessment and intervention sessions can be appropriately structured. Ignorance of individual differences and levels of acculturation can ultimately result in an inappropriate and, perhaps, offensive approach to the inter action (Anderson and Battle, 1993; Cheng, 1993; Bebout and Arthur, 1992; Chan, 1992; Cheng, 1989a; Matsuda, 1989). Similarly, believing that all members of one cultural group assume the same values, attitudes and practices is inappropriate. Cultural differences exist from one family to another, as well as culture to culture.

Case example

Jorge is a 40-year-old roofer recently injured on the job. It was his first day of his work hardening programme and he was scheduled to be evaluated by the occupational therapist (OT) at 10:00 a.m. The OT was planning on administering some standardised assessments and interviewing him. She was informed that Jorge did not speak English the day before the session, and had to arrange for a Spanish interpreter to come in the following day. Jorge arrived at 9:40 a.m. and someone from the staff pointed him in the direction of the OT department. The OT smiled and in her limited Spanish tried to tell him that the interpreter would not be there until 10:00 a.m. Jorge seemed nervous and was looking around a lot. The OT offered him some coffee or something to drink, but he shook his head and told her something in Spanish that she did not understand. She smiled awkwardly and pointed to the clock. He smiled back, but still appeared somewhat anxious. Finally, the interpreter arrived at 9:55 a.m.

The interpreter introduced herself to the OT and Jorge. Jorge seemed a little bit more relaxed. The interpreter asked the OT where the bathroom was located because Jorge would like to use it. She then realised that was probably what he was trying to say to her earlier. The OT did not have much time, but she gave the interpreter a quick, brief rundown on her plans for the session. The interpreter started to tell her that she was not familiar with occupational therapy as Jorge returned from the bathroom. The OT realised that she needed to get started or she would run out of time.

The OT started the session and she tried to remember to pause to allow for interpretation. The interpreter was doing her best to keep up with the OT, but was often asking her to repeat what she said. At times during the session the OT was speaking very loudly. She looked at the interpreter while she was talking throughout the session and really did not have a lot of eye contact with Jorge. The OT asked Jorge to pick up a box and asked him if he had any pain right now. He nodded, but he continued to lift the box. The OT was confused because Jorge did not look as if he was in pain and he was lifting the box without a lot of effort. The OT wanted to ask the interpreter a question about this, but was not sure when the appropriate time to interrupt her was, so she did not say anything. As the session progressed, the interpreter seemed to be doing all the interacting with Jorge and the OT faded into the background. Nonetheless at this point in time the OT was just trying to get the information she needed and was concerned about running over the scheduled time.

> The OT ended the session because the interpreter was expected somewhere else and she had another client waiting. The OT was not able to get as much information as she would have like to and she did not feel satisfied with the level of interaction between her and Jorge. Anyhow, she thanked Jorge and told him that she would see him tomorrow at the same time.
>
> (Ruiz, 1996, p. 44)

There are a number of factors that have influenced the success of this session. Overall, the session was not very successful. The occupational therapist was unable to gather the information she needed, the session was rushed, and it seems as if little rapport was achieved between the patient and clinician. Although an interpreter was used to bridge the linguistic and cultural gap between the OT and Jorge, several barriers developed to impede the process of the interaction.

Last-minute notification of the need to arrange an interpreter. In any workplace environment, procedures need to be in place to ensure that the patient's interpreting needs are identified as early as possible. This will allow for an interpreter to be arranged earlier (important when there is a high demand on interpreting services or when interpreting services are limited and alternative arrangements need to be made). It will also allow time for the clinician to begin the process of culture learning through familiarization with some of the common features of the patient's language and/or culture. If the clinician is inexperienced in working with an interpreter, it will also allow more time for researching some of the important points in conducting an interpreted session.

Inadequate pre-session briefing with the interpreter due to time constraints. Thus, there was little opportunity to discuss . . .

- The clinician's experience working with interpreters and the interpreter's experience working with occupational therapists.
- The goals of the session. Making interpreters aware of what you hope to achieve during the session will provide them with some insight into your assessment procedures and will guide their judgement of how best to interpret for your purposes.
- Assessment procedures and materials. Most standardized assessment tools are based on the dominant culture in which the test was developed and may, therefore, consist of culturally biased stimuli questions or materials and will have culture- and language-specific norms. The pre-session briefing can be used to discuss the relevance and appropriateness of particular testing materials and/or questions for the patient's language and

cultural background. It will also give the interpreter time to prepare any questions that require careful interpretation.

- Roles and needs of the interpreter and clinician. Taking the time to discuss this can avoid some of the frustrating incidents that occurred in the session with Jorge, such as not knowing whether to look at the patient or the interpreter, losing control of the session, losing (or never establishing) rapport with the patient, not knowing how or when to interrupt or request clarification, speaking too fast or too loud, and not knowing when to pause for interpretation. This is particularly important when either or both parties have limited experience working with the other profession.

- How problems are to be addressed and resolved. It can be particularly important to discuss options for repairing potential or actual breakdowns in the interaction. For example, methods for requesting clarification or repetition, methods for gathering further information about the patient's culture/language/background that may affect the communication process, methods for repairing a message that may be culturally insensitive/inappropriate or linguistically ambiguous and difficult to interpret, and so on.

Unrealistic time expectations.

- It cannot be assumed or expected that interpreter-mediated sessions will achieve the same goals in the same amount of time as an ordinary session. As a general rule it should be assumed that everything will take at least twice as long. An extended session or multiple sessions may be required to gather the same amount of information normally achieved in one session.

Lack of eye contact with the patient.

- An interpreted session is in every other way the same as an ordinary same-language session. The interaction between the clinician and patient should only be altered to suit the cultural characteristics of the patient (for example, it may be recommended that prolonged direct eye contact be avoided as much as possible as this may be seen by the patient as a sign of disrespect or hostility). The patient is still your patient and deserves your attention and direct interaction, as much as possible within the bounds of appropriate behaviour for the patient's culture. Failing to interact with the patient directly may serve to:
  - impede the establishment or development of rapport;
  - direct more power and control of the session to the interpreter;
  - alienate the patient.

Cultural discrepancy between the patient and interpreter.

- Although the interpreter and Jorge were both Spanish-speaking, they came from different backgrounds. In the above example, when the occupational therapist asked if Jorge was feeling any pain now when lifting the box, the word the interpreter used for 'now' may have meant 'later' to Jorge, as it does in some regions where Spanish is spoken (Ruiz, 1996). This sort of difficulty may be prevented by finding out the region or country patients come from or, if appropriate, which dialect they speak, and then arranging a matching interpreter.

No time for post-session debriefing with the interpreter to discuss:

- cultural issues;
- overall impressions of the session and assessment results;
- problems identified (for example, incongruency between Jorge's report of pain on lifting the box without physical evidence of discomfort; knowing when and how to request clarification; speaking rate, and so forth);
- preparation for next session.

The example of Jorge and the occupational therapist provides a useful insight into the potential difficulties that can occur in an interpreter-mediated session, especially when one or both parties have limited awareness of the goals, procedures, and requirements of the session and the experiences, needs, and roles of the other professional. Thus, barriers to communication may arise when:

- the *purpose* of the interaction is not fully understood by either party;
- the clinician does not have a developed sense of intercultural issues;
- the suitability of the interaction style, and/or session activities, is not discussed;
- the needs of the interpreter and the needs of the clinician are not discussed in sufficient detail or at all.

Food for thought

Using the session you previously described as unsatisfactory (Activity 6.1), revise your reasons why the session did not work according to plan. Consider how you and the interpreter may have influenced the session.

CHAPTER 9

Models of partnership

During any interaction, an interpreter may assume a variety of roles. Which role is chosen depends upon the needs of the interaction at that point in time. Faust and Drickey (1986) identified four roles of an interpreter:

*   interviewer;
*   instrument of the clinician;
*   client advocate;
*   culture broker.

As an interviewer, the interpreter works as the main communicative partner with the client, receiving guidance from the clinician about what sort of information to collect from the client and then reporting back to the clinician when the requested information has been gathered. In a speech-language pathology session, an interpreter may be used in this way to assess a patient's communication skills by asking questions from a sheet provided by the clinician. As an instrument of the clinician, the interpreter remains under the controlled guidance of the clinician and may be expected to interpret all information word for word. As a client advocate, the interpreter is able to freely provide the client or clinician with any additional information he or she feels is important for them to know, or to ask questions on behalf of the client, without direction from either party. Finally, as a culture broker, the interpreter acts a mediator of cultural differences (Faust and Drickey, 1986).

Within the context of SLP, there is an opening to expand the fourth role of the interpreter to include the provision of information about the patient's language. This modified role could be termed *cultural and linguistic informant*. Faust and Drickey (1986) propose a model of the inter-relationship between the clinician (provider), patient and interpreter, called the 'PPI triangle'. The model demonstrates the triangular relationship between the three participants in any interpreter-mediated interaction. All partners have direct access to the others, although the link between the clinician (provider) and the patient can only act on a non-verbal level. Faust and Drickey (1986) propose that an understanding of this model would allow clinicians to actively guide the interaction so that the interpreter assumes the role that is most appropriate to the interaction at a particular point in time.

As a model of partnership between the clinician and interpreter, Faust and Drickey's PPI triangle has several advantages. First, it identifies and embraces the collaborative nature of the interpretation process. It is flexible, allowing for the roles to change within a single interaction and it accounts for communication on both verbal and non-verbal levels. Lastly, it hints at the need for the clinician to be aware of the interpreter's roles and needs so that effective use of the partnership can be achieved.

However, there are some limitations. One is that this model only seems to provide a superficial overview of the relationship between the clinician and interpreter, without expanding on how a collaborative partnership can be achieved or maintained. Three of the roles identified by Faust and Drickey (1986) seem to represent extremes in the relationship between the participants in the interaction. That is, interpreters act for themselves (interviewer), for the client (client advocate), or for the clinician (instrument of the clinician) exclusively. In addition, the model seems to promote the way in which the clinician can control the movement of the interpreter's role, rather than promoting a joint control of this. Finally, and perhaps most importantly, the model does not identify the roles of the clinician in the partnership.

The collaborative partnership model

In the collaborative partnership model (Figure 9.3) the roles of the interpreter are as described by Faust and Drickey (1986), with some modifications:

- instrument of the clinician;
- client advocate;
- cultural and linguistic informant (as opposed to culture broker);
- independent actor (expanded from interviewer to allow the interpreter to request or provide information about the session/interpretation/roles/ skills, and so forth, and keeping with the aim to promote shared knowledge and clear communication so as to enhance the interpretation process).

As previously mentioned, these roles seem to represent extremes, and we can now place them on continua plotting degree of control and supply of information (Figure 9.1).

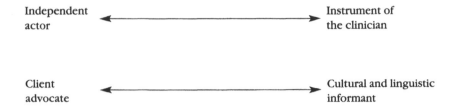

Figure 9.1. The roles of the interpreter, plotted along continua.

The 'independent actor — instrument of the clinician' continuum represents control over the interaction. At one extreme (independent actor), the interpreter assumes the majority of control over the interaction, acting independently to gather or provide information as he or she sees fit. At the other extreme (instrument of the clinician), the interpreter acts under the controlled and full guidance of the clinician.

The 'client advocate — cultural and linguistic informant' continuum represents the supply of information during the interaction (including pre- and post-session discussions). At one extreme (client advocate), the interpreter acts on behalf of the client, providing or gathering information to help him or her gain the most benefit from the assessment or treatment session. At the other extreme (cultural and linguistic informant), the interpreter acts on behalf of the clinician, providing information of a cultural or linguistic nature which may influence the processes or procedures used in the session.

In keeping with a collaborative partnership theme, the roles of the clinician also need to be identified. These can be described as:

- Observer — the clinician assumes a passive role, observing the interaction between, and behaviours of, the other participants.
- Controller — the clinician assumes the highest degree of control over the interaction and input or behaviours of the others, especially the interpreter.
- Process informant — the clinician provides the interpreter, and patient/carer, with information about the session, goals, procedures, and roles.
- Instrument of the interpreter — the clinician's behaviour is guided by the interpreter.

These roles also represent extremes, and can be plotted along continua, as in Figure 9.2. As with the roles of the interpreter, these also represent degree of control and supply of information.

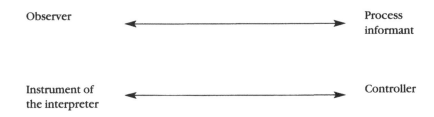

Figure 9.2. The roles of the speech-language pathologist, plotted along continua.

The 'observer — process informant' continuum represents the supply of information during the interaction, so that the clinician can either choose to provide information or passively observe, at any point in time. The 'instrument of the interpreter — controller' continuum represents the degree of control exercised by the clinician, so that at any point in time the clinician can exercise full control over the behaviour of the interpreter or be guided by the interpreter in the behaviours and session procedures they choose to use.

The roles of the interpreter and the roles of the clinician are interrelated and their continua are plotted on the same diagram to show how they work together to achieve collaborative partnership (Figure 9.3).

By plotting all four continua together, it can be seen that the most collaborative partnership is achieved when the interpreter and clinician borrow a little from all their roles. That is, when information and control is shared. Once a collaborative partnership has been established, it is possible for there to be movement outside the bounds of the inner circle, so that the interpreter or clinician assumes or surrenders more control, and provides or withholds more information. This movement is negotiated during the collaboration process and depends upon the needs of the interaction at any point in time, given the aim to gather the most accurate and appropriate information from the client for assessment or intervention purposes. This model stresses the need for SLPs and interpreters to be aware of each other's roles, to share information, and work together to provide the patient with the best possible service.

Case example

Natalie is a speech-language pathologist working in a community health setting. She has an initial assessment at 10 o'clock this morning of Lucy, a three-year-old girl of Vietnamese-speaking background. She received the referral from Lucy's medical practitioner some weeks ago, but was only able to schedule an interpreter for today. Knowing that interpreted sessions normally take more time, Natalie has allowed herself the rest of the morning

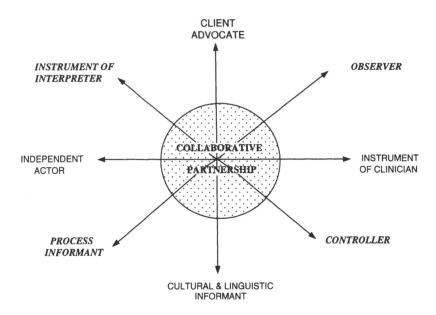

Figure 9.3. The collaborative partnership model for interpreter-mediated interactions. The roles of the interpreter and clinician (italics) are shown on continua.

to complete the assessment. She has arranged the interpreter to arrive at 9:45 a.m. for a pre-session discussion, and has booked her for one and a half hours, allowing for one hour of assessment and 15 minutes each of briefing and debriefing before and after the session (time management). Having had some weeks prior to the appointment, Natalie revised some of the main cultural and linguistic features of Vietnamese that may affect her assessment procedure (culture learning).

The interpreter arrived just before 9:50 a.m. It was an interpreter Natalie had worked with twice before on initial assessments, so she knew she would not need to go into as much detail about the assessment procedures. Instead Natalie briefly described what she was planning to do in terms of interview questions, informal assessment approaches, and what aspects of Lucy's speech and language she needed the interpreter to look out for (process informant). Mai, the interpreter, clarified her role with Natalie and questioned her more specifically about some of the assessment activities (independent actor). Natalie (instrument of the interpreter and process informant) then discussed with Mai (cultural and linguistic informant) the cultural and linguistic features of Vietnamese that may affect the assessment outcomes or interaction with Lucy or her mother. Procedures for addressing any potential breakdowns in communication during the session were negotiated and the session goals quickly revised (Natalie: process informant, controller, instrument of interpreter; Mai: instrument of the clinician, independent actor).

Lucy and her mother arrived for the appointment. Natalie and Mai went out together to greet them and introduce themselves. In the clinic room, Mai briefly explained the roles of each professional and what the appointment was *for* (client advocate) and then she explained to Natalie what she had said (independent actor). Natalie began the assessment by interviewing Lucy's mother (controller) and Mai interpreted everything that was said (instrument of the clinician). At one point in time, Mai noticed that Lucy's mother had not understood the question Natalie had asked. She explained this to Natalie (independent actor) and suggested that she explain why she needs to ask that question in case Lucy's mother does not understand the relevance of it, given a different cultural view about the causes of illness/disability (cultural and linguistic informant).

The interview was completed and Natalie moved onto the floor to play with Lucy. Mai also moved onto the floor to be involved in the interaction, as negotiated prior to the session. Natalie watched the interaction between Mai and Lucy for a short time (observer) allowing them to establish some rapport. Then she began her informal assessment of Lucy's speech and language (controller). At each activity Natalie briefly reminded Mai about the purpose of the task and what to look out for (process informant). Mai interpreted Natalie's comments and instructions to Lucy, and Lucy's utterances/responses back to Natalie, including a description of any unusual features (instrument of the clinician). During the assessment, Natalie noticed that Lucy was having particular difficulty responding to her questions and instructions involving a book about a holiday to the seaside. She discussed this with Mai and Lucy's mother, as she thought that Lucy may not be familiar with this sort of book or theme (Natalie: instrument of the interpreter, process informant; Mai: client advocate, instrument of the clinician, cultural and linguistic informant).

At the end of the assessment, Natalie discussed her findings with Lucy's mother, and suggested options for intervention (controller). Mai interpreted everything said (instrument of the clinician), and both she and Natalie watched out for any problems or breakdowns in communication (Natalie: observer; Mai: client advocate, independent actor).

After Lucy and her mother had left, Natalie and Mai had 20 minutes to discuss any issues that were observed during the session but were not addressed at the time, including issues relating to Lucy's performance, cultural and linguistic features influencing the interaction, the interpretation process, and the working partnership between themselves (Natalie: controller, process informant, instrument of the interpreter; Mai: cultural and linguistic informant, independent actor, instrument of the clinician).

Natalie and Mai had established an understanding of each other's roles and needs from the very beginning of the interaction, setting up an avenue for the sharing of information, clear communication, negotiation, and mutual respect for how each could help the other. The pre-session discussion was instrumental in allowing the time for this partnership to develop. The session consequently ran smoothly, and although there were a number of potential problems with interview questions and assessment techniques, Mai's awareness of the session goals and Natalie's awareness of cultural and linguistic differences meant that these problems were identified and addressed. This sort of mutual understanding in professional roles and needs can only serve to improve the interactions we have with our patients, resulting in better practice and outcomes.

Activity 9.1

Using the session you previously described as unsatisfactory (Activity 6.1), identify the ways in which you can facilitate an improved working partnership with the interpreter and achieve better outcomes for your assessment or intervention.

Reflecting back on the interpreter-mediated session you previously described as less than satisfactory (Activity 6.1), you may have identified the following points as ways to facilitate an improved working partnership with the interpreter and therefore achieve better outcomes from your session:

- improved time management;
- allowing additional time to achieve what you would normally achieve in a similar same-language session;
- planning time for pre-session briefing (10 minutes of pre-session briefing can save much time in the long run and contribute to a smooth flowing session in which you achieve your goals and gather the information you need);
- planning time for post-session debriefing (this may or may not be needed, but it is important to allow the time for it in case there are specific issues which need to be discussed prior to the next session, to clarify information gathered, for example);
- improving your knowledge on how to work with interpreters;
- talking with colleagues, discussing their experiences and listening to their advice;
- reading relevant literature;
- talking with the interpreter service — they may have brochures or information booklets available that outline the roles and qualifications of their interpreters and include information on how best to work with an interpreter;

- attending training sessions, if available;
- investigating relevant aspects of your patient's language and culture;
- talking with local cultural groups — if available, these groups may have information outlining some of the main characteristics of the patient's language and culture;
- reading relevant literature;
- talking with the interpreter, particularly regarding language and cultural influences on specific aspects of your session;
- reducing your level of anxiety;
- improving your knowledge on how to work with interpreters;
- being open to alternative ways of being (broad categorizing and uncertainty oriented);
- investigating relevant aspects of the patient's language and culture;
- discussing methods for addressing communication breakdowns prior to the session;
- explaining professional jargon to promote more accurate interpretation;
- using shorter, less complex sentence forms that might be easier to interpret;
- arranging for a professionally trained interpreter, if available, being sure to match for language and culture, and, if appropriate, age and gender;
- if only untrained interpreters are available, being sure that their language and culture match those of the patient, that their language and cultural knowledge is adequate, that they understand your role and aims of the session, that their gender, age, or relationship to the patient will not have a negative affect on the success of the session.

You may have identified other points, more specific to your own experiences, in addition to or instead of the above. The importance of an exercise such as this is being able to reflect on and analyse your experiences, so that you can identify ways to improve your work style in the light of the information discussed in this book.

Making it work

When faced with the challenge of communicating interculturally and via an interpreter, a number of options are open to us. Professional interpreters who, ideally, are trained in health-care interpreting and who are competently bilingual and bicultural (or multilingual and multicultural as the case may be) should be chosen over untrained interpreters such as bilingual staff, family members or friends. However, there are many situations in which it is not possible to access professionally trained interpreters and, therefore, family members, bilingual staff or friends must be called upon to bridge the communication and cultural gap. We have discussed the complexities of intercultural communication competence and we identified the need to develop our own awareness of other cultures and the existence of alternate interpretations of behaviour (that is, to be broad catergorizers and uncertainty oriented). This is especially important in situations where untrained interpreters need to be used, as a greater awareness of the cultural and linguistic influences on behaviour will allow more flexible evaluation of the partnership formed with the interpreter. This can have the effect of alerting us to potential problems in the interpretation process in terms of the patient's/carer's or interpreter's behaviour. As there are many factors that can cause difficulties when working with untrained interpreters, when entering into this situation, clinicians should consider the following questions:

- Will the interpreter remain neutral in the interaction or will he or she be biased by his or her own cultural influences and/or personal beliefs?
- How competent is the interpreter in the languages of the patient and clinician?
- How competent is the interpreter in his or her knowledge of both cultures?
- Does using the chosen interpreter disrupt family or social roles (for example using a daughter to interpret for an elderly man)?
- How much does the interpreter know about the clinician's discipline or about interpreting in a health-care context?
- Does the clinician have the time to educate the interpreter about the purpose and needs of the session before the session begins?
- Does the interpreter have the time to be educated by the clinician?
- Does the interpreter have the knowledge of how to interpret the information as accurately as possible for the needs of the session?
- Does the clinician have the knowledge of how to discuss interpreting styles (including strategies for repair) with the interpreter so that they gather the most accurate information?
- Does the clinician explain jargon terms so that they are unambiguous and easily translatable?

A partnership should be achieved with any interpreter but when using untrained interpreters the clinician needs to work harder to establish the skills of the interpreter, to be aware of potential difficulties and possible solutions, and to establish an effective rapport with the interpreter. In doing so, it is vitally important for clinicians to understand the complexity of the interpretation process, understand and respect the skills of the interpreter, exercise flexibility in sharing control, and recognize the need to inform the interpreter of the aims, goals, and procedures of the session.

Effective time management is essential. Interpreted sessions will always take longer, not just because of the need for all information to be repeated but because of the complex cultural and linguistic issues that may influence your assessment or treatment approach. Scheduling enough time for a relaxed and collaborative pre-session briefing with the interpreter will ultimately:

- reduce the amount of time wasted on communication breakdowns (resolved or unresolved);
- reduce the amount of time spent chasing up and clarifying ambiguous information;
- reduce anxiety by knowing that you and the interpreter are working together to achieve the same goal; and
- result in a more satisfying session, with better outcomes for the patient.

Before any session involving a patient from a cultural or linguistic background different from your own it will be important to consider the session in a holistic way, thinking about your own behaviours and attitudes, as well as those of the patient and interpreter (if one is required) and how these may influence your interaction and your session goals and procedures. The following questions may be useful in helping you to determine what needs to be considered when planning an intercultural or interpreter-mediated session:

- How has culture influenced your own communication and interaction style, including the assessment and treatment approaches you use?
- What are your feelings, including fears and anxieties about this session?
- How can you develop your skills to become uncertainty oriented and a broad categorizer?
- Where can you gather information about this patient's language and culture?
- What information will you need to know about the patient before the session?
- What information will you need to know about the patient's culture before the session?
- What information will you need to know about the patient's language before the session?
- What assessment or treatment approach are you planning to use?
- Is it culturally appropriate?
- How will you use the results?
- Who else will you gather information from?
- What will be your back-up plan in case this approach does not work as you expect?

- If an interpreter is needed, are the activity questions/stimuli items easy to interpret?
- If an interpreter is needed, what time will you give them to become familiar with testing or treatment items?
- If any material requires translation (written), what time will you give the interpreter to do this?
- Have you allowed enough time to achieve all your goals and tasks?
- Have you allowed time for pre- and post-session discussions with the interpreter?
- What information will you provide the interpreter before the session?
- What information will you gather from the interpreter before the session?
- How will you modify your communication style to suit interpretation and intercultural communication?
- How will potential or actual miscommunications be dealt with during the session?
- What information will you discuss with the interpreter after the session?

CHAPTER 10

Future directions

It is hoped that this book has stirred (or renewed) interest in developing services for patients from culturally and linguistically diverse populations, whatever your clinical setting. This is an ever-increasing field of practice. Yet, in the discipline of speech-language pathology there has been relatively little research and literature giving consideration to multicultural perspectives in clinical practice. Literature reviewing research and clinical cases reported in other disciplines is useful and can be applied to SLP practice. However, our professional field is unique and there are many specific questions that need to be answered before we can truly admit to embracing cultural and linguistic diversity within our services. We have certainly raised our awareness of the important issues in recent years but we still have a long way to go. Research is needed in SLP to substantiate the (probably valid) assumptions we often make about our clinical procedures and policies. It would probably not be an overstatement to suggest that many SLPs have their own clinical tools and procedures for assessing or treating patients from cultural and linguistic minority backgrounds, including modified tests, stimuli items, case history questionnaires, as well as a range of service policies (for example, for accessibility, equity, managing non-attendance, service evaluation, community liaison, and so on). In addition, it would probably be fair to say that the majority of these policies and resources were developed at an individual clinician or service level and have not been clinically trialled or widely distributed. If this is the case, then we are sitting on a mountain of research opportunity for both clinical and managerial aspects of SLP services. We should be working together, sharing our knowledge and resources, through publications, research, and interest groups that can be widely (ideally internationally) accessible.

Our research needs encompass the broad spectrum of multicultural issues for SLP, including cultural influences on communication, multicultural speech-language pathology from service level and clinical perspectives, interpreter-mediated SLP, and undergraduate education. Boxes 10.1 to 10.5 offer some suggestions for research opportunities in these five areas.

Box 10.1. Cultural influences on communication

- The extent and type of miscommunication during SLP sessions (same language context). This and the following areas have the potential to be further subdivided to focus on specific aspects of a session, such as case history interview, patient/parent feedback and therapy activities.
- Causes of miscommunication during SLP sessions.
- Impact of non-verbal communication. Implications of cultural difference on SLP sessions.
- Strategies for improving communication in same language, different cultural encounters in SLP.
- Communicating with professional colleagues from culturally diverse backgrounds.
- SLP knowledge of cultural influences on communication and implications for clinical practice.

Box 10.2. Intercultural speech-language pathology — service level

- SLP: the culture of our profession.
- Service delivery: are management strategies to reduce waiting lists culturally equitable?
- Perception of SLP in non-mainstream cultures.
- Education opportunities and needs for SLPs managing culturally and linguistically diverse patient populations.
- Managing cultural and linguistic diversity in SLP practice: review of service policies.
- Availability of and need for patient/family support services.

Education of qualified SLPs and undergraduate students is the key to improving the cultural competence of our profession. Preliminary results from SLPs who attended a training workshop as part of my research study show a strong correlation between education and subsequent knowledge and perceived skill, as well as decreased levels of anxiety and uncertainty, in managing patients from culturally and linguistically diverse populations and in working with interpreters (Isaac, 2001c). However, the preliminary results also suggest a correlation between some content areas in the training programme. For example, awareness of cultural influences on communication and session procedures seems to underlie knowledge and perceived skill about the type of information to share with an interpreter prior to an assessment/therapy session. This is not really surprising given the intricate nature of intercultural and interpreter-mediated communication. However,

---

Box 10.3. Intercultural speech-language pathology — clinical

- Anxiety and uncertainty in SLPs working with culturally and linguistically diverse populations.
- Patient-professional roles: expectations, cultural differences, strategies.
- Non-attendance and non-compliance: what do they really reflect?
- Strategies for managing non-attendance and non-compliance in cultural and linguistic minority groups.
- Perceptions of communication disorder — causes, treatment, and expected outcomes.
- Culturally focused case history information — what to find out, how, when, and with whom: implications for assessment outcomes.
- Patient/family satisfaction following assessment. Traditional versus culturally focused approach.
- Culturally focused assessment methods — case studies, comparisons, clinical trials.
- Developing assessment tools for patients of bilingual background.
- Patient/family satisfaction with treatment approach.
- Culturally focused treatment methods — case studies, comparisons, clinical trials.
- Liaison between SLP and other significant agencies in the management of culturally and linguistically diverse patient populations (for example, school, ESL/LEP support programmes, medical staff, allied health staff, multidisciplinary teams, community leaders in the patient's cultural group).
- Communication characteristics of ESL/LEP children referred for SLP assessment/management.

---

it does strongly suggest that training programmes need to be holistic. They need to address the issues with minimal assumption about participants' background knowledge. There may be little value in offering a seminar or workshop on establishing partnerships with interpreters if participants lack the background knowledge about the influence of cultural and linguistic differences on communication and assessment/therapy procedures.

In undergraduate education the pedagogical issue is whether to teach cultural and linguistic diversity in SLP as a core subject in its own right or to address clinical and managerial issues as they arise throughout other subjects, such as addressing culturally focused assessment as part of the core subject on child speech and language disorders, or addressing bilingual aphasia as part of a subject on adult neurological disorders. If managing cultural and linguistic diversity is regarded as a core subject in its own right

---

Box 10.4. Interpreter-mediated speech-language pathology

- Accessibility of trained versus untrained interpreters.
- Use of trained versus untrained interpreters in the clinical context.
- Education opportunities and needs of SLPs working with interpreters.
- Education opportunities and needs of interpreters working with SLPs.
- Difficulties arising from interpretation in clinical scenarios.
- Sharing knowledge: pre-session briefing between SLPs and interpreters.
- Implications of pre-session briefing for assessment outcomes and SLP/interpreter satisfaction.
- Patient/family satisfaction following interpreter-mediated sessions.
- SLP knowledge of interpreter skills and roles.
- Impact of education on SLP knowledge for working with interpreters.
- Anxiety and uncertainty in SLPs working with interpreters.
- Impact of education on SLPs' anxiety and uncertainty in working with interpreters.

Box 10.5. Undergraduate education

- Training opportunities and needs for SLP students in managing cultural and linguistic diversity.
- Recommendations for core content in training programmes.
- Opportunity to develop clinical skills with patients from cultural and linguistic minority groups: recommendations for clinical practice experiences.
- Clinical educators' abilities to provide effective learning experiences with patients from cultural and linguistic minority groups.
- Pedagogical issues: should multicultural SLP be a core subject in its own right? Should it be addressed across existing SLP core subjects as the opportunity arises? Or a combination of both?

---

then it may be most suitable to address the issues across all years in the undergraduate programme, matching content to the general course outline for each year. For example, exploring issues related to intercultural communication and miscommunication early in the course while moving on to advanced issues, such as designing augmentative/alternate communication systems for culturally and linguistically diverse patient populations or working with families of children with special needs (for example those with cerebral palsy) in a later year. Teaching the subject as an intensive final year course has the advantage of keeping students focused on managing cultural and linguistic diversity from basic to advanced topics, however it may minimize the opportunity for students to explore their knowledge and skills in genuine clinical learning experiences throughout their undergraduate programme.

In many cases the approach chosen will reflect the philosophy of the teaching institution or undergraduate programme. However, it may not always represent the best choice for the students or the profession. Perhaps the value of education in this area, as well as the relative merits of different teaching approaches, need to be explored so that academic staff have a case to argue for pedagogical change. Similarly, a useful place to start, perhaps, would be cross-institution discussion on the advantages and disadvantages of the various teaching approaches being used, including content and opportunity for practical experience.

Practical experience in managing cultural and linguistic diversity would have to be regarded as a key element in students' development of cultural competence. Clinical practice placements which allow students to explore a variety of service delivery models for patients from cultural and linguistic minority groups, practice assessment and intervention skills, and work with interpreters, would serve to reinforce students' theoretical knowledge. However, it is vital for clinical educators to be cognizant with the issues surrounding cultural and linguistic diversity in patient management and to be able to effectively teach those skills to students. It may be valuable for prospective clinical educators to attend a workshop to receive information about the undergraduate course content, philosophy, and expectations of clinical experience. In addition to coursework time it may be useful for students to have the opportunity to attend small-group tutorials to discuss specific issues relating to their clinical placement experiences in an informal forum.

Recruiting bilingual students into undergraduate training programmes for speech-language pathology may be one solution to the challenges of managing cultural and linguistic diversity in clinical practice. However, there are some areas that should be considered before bilingual students (and, therefore, bilingual SLPs) are 'labelled' as specialists in a particular language group. In Chapter 6 it was argued that the process of interpretation required bilingual and *bicultural* competence. This same argument can be applied to bilingual SLPs — for effective and appropriate assessment and intervention of culturally and linguistically diverse patient populations, the SLP should ideally be bilingual as well as bicultural. The enormous influence culture has on all aspects of communication, including non-verbal features, does not need to be restated. In addition, culture and language are dynamic and susceptible to influence from other cultural groups and languages. Thus, a student whose non-English exposures have been limited to minority group experiences within an English-language society may have language and cultural knowledge and skills that do not exactly match the language or cultural experiences of patients who have native proficiency. Despite these potential problems, bilingual proficiency is a desirable characteristic for SLPs working with culturally and linguistically diverse patient populations. However, it may be unwise to assume that bilingual students or SLPs do not require support in developing their knowledge and skills in effective management of patients from non-English-speaking backgrounds. In contrast, support in the form of specific training programmes may help these students and professionals to identify potential limitations in their knowledge/skill base while sharing clinical management ideas.

In the culture of best practice and quality management we have a professional responsibility to ensure that the service we provide to patients from cultural and linguistic minority groups is of the highest standard. We must ask ourselves 'Are our services working at their most effective and efficient levels?' Limited knowledge and skill for managing cultural and linguistic diversity for communication disorders may result in:

- wasted time for the professionals involved, the service, and the patient;
- wasted money for the professionals involved, the service, and the patient;
- an overall dissatisfaction with the service provided, including feelings of distrust;
- inadequate gathering of information during assessment;
- misdiagnosis based on inadequate, incomplete or inaccurate information;
- inappropriate intervention goals;
- inappropriate intervention approach;
- patient non-compliance and/or non-attendance;
- slow or no progress through intervention;
- frustration;
- inappropriate patient discharge based on personal judgement that the patient is non-compliant or not interested in continuing intervention.

The ethical implications of these potential scenarios are clear. Speech-language pathologists must take responsibility for their patients' management and their own professional conduct. Gentile, Ozolins, and Vasilakakos (1996, p. 14) discuss the use of untrained interpreters and the risk of serious communication breakdown when family members, friends, or other bilingual helpers are used. They suggest that there is a developing recognition of the 'serious breach of ethics on the part of the professional, official, or worker from any institution that has to deal with speakers of a minority language' that can occur when untrained interpreters are used. Developing cultural competence through education and research will help professionals to effectively evaluate their services, and themselves, and reach for new heights in clinical management. Good enough is probably not enough. Best practice is the ideal, but more research and collaboration is needed to develop and expand on guidelines for improved service delivery and clinical management.

Concluding thoughts

If this book were a sea and you were a swimmer amongst its pages, I wonder whether you would imagine yourself being tossed about by crashing waves of cultural reality or whether you would imagine yourself drifting on the tide towards cultural competence. Either way I hope that I have made you aware of the intricacies and delicacies of managing cultural and linguistic diversity for communication disorders. Developing a culturally focused service can be a long and arduous task, especially if your current work practices leave you with many unanswered questions. Yet, your efforts will be richly rewarded and your service will be more effective, more efficient, and more valuable to yourself, your profession, and, most importantly, your patients.

References

Anderson NB, Battle DE (1993) Cultural diversity in the development of language. In DE Battle (ed.) Communication Disorders in Multicultural Populations. Boston: Andover Medical Publishers, pp. 158-85.

Anderson RT (1998) Examining language loss in bilingual children. Multicultural Electronic Journal of Communication Disorders [online] 1(1). At http://www.asha. ucf.edu/languagearticles.html.

Baker NG (1981) Social work through an interpreter. Social Work 26: 391-7.

Barnett S (1989) Working with interpreters. In DM Duncan (ed.) Working with Bilingual Language Disability. London: Chapman & Hall, pp. 91-112.

Battle DE (ed.) (1993) Communication Disorders in Multicultural Populations. Boston: Andover Medical Publishers.

Bebout L, Arthur B (1992) Cross-cultural attitudes towards speech disorders. Journal of Speech and Hearing Research 35: 45-52.

Benton AL, Hamsher K deS, Sivan AB (1994) Multilingual Aphasia Examination (3 edn). Iowa City: AJA Associates.

Boehm AE (1971) The Boehm Test of Basic Concepts. New York: Psychological Corporation.

Brownell R (1987) Receptive one-word picture vocabulary test: Upper extension. Novato CA: Academic Therapy.

Buchwald D, Caralis PV, Gany F, Hardt EJ, Muecke MA, Putsch RW (1993) The medical interview across cultures. Patient Care, April 15, 141-66.

Burt M, Dulay H, Hernandez-Chavez E (1978) Bilingual Syntax Measure. New York: Harcourt Brace Jovanovich.

Carrow E (1973) Test for Auditory Comprehension of Language. Allen TX: DLM Teaching Resources.

Carrow E (1974) Austin Spanish Articulation Test. Hingham MA: Teaching Resources.

Chan S (1992) Families with Asian roots. In EW Lynch and MJ Hanson (eds) Developing Cross-cultural Competence: A guide for working with young children and their families. Baltimore: PH Brookes, pp. 181-257.

Cheng LL (1989a) Service delivery to Asian/Pacific LEP children: a cross-cultural framework. Topics in Language Disorders 9(3): 1-14.

Cheng LL (1989b) Intervention strategies: a multicultural approach. Topics in Language Disorders 9(3): 84-91.

Cheng LL (1991) Assessing Asian Language Performance: Guidelines for evaluating limited-English-proficient students. Oceanside: Academic Communication Associates.

Cheng LL (1993) Asian-American cultures. In DE Battle (ed.) Communication Disorders in Multicultural Populations. Boston: Andover Medical Publishers, pp. 38-77.

Cheng LL (1996) Beyond bilingualism: a quest for communicative competence. Topics in Language Disorders 16(4): 9-21.

Cheng LL (1997) Diversity: challenges and implications for assessment. Journal of Children's Communication Development 19(1) 53-61.

Costello Ingham J (1993) Behavioural treatment of stuttering children. In R Curlee (ed.) Stuttering and Related Disorders of Fluency. New York: Thieme, pp 68-100.

Cummins J (1984) Bilingualism and Special Education: Issues in assessment and pedagogy. Clevedon: Multilingual Matters.

DeAvila E, Duncan SE (1983) Language Assessment Scales. Monterey CA: CTB/McGraw Hill.

Delbar V (1999) From the desert: transcultural aspects of cancer nursing care in Israel. Cancer Nursing 22: 45-51.

Dentino AN (1991) Letter to the editor. Hospital and Community Psychiatry 42: 858.

Diaz-Duque OF (1982) Overcoming the language barrier: advice from an interpreter. American Journal of Nursing, September 1380-2.

Dunn LM, Lugo DE, Padilla ER, Dunn LM (1986) Test de Vocabulario en Imagines Peabody. Circle Pines MN: American Guidance Service.

Faust S, Drickey R (1986) Working with interpreters. The Journal of Family Practice 22: 131-8.

Freimanis C (1994) Training bilinguals to interpret in the community. In RW Brislin, T Yoshida (eds) Improving Intercultural Interactions: Modules for cross-cultural training programs. London: Sage Publications, pp. 313-41.

Frey R, Roberts-Smith L, Bessell-Browne S (eds) (1990) Working with Interpreters in Law, Health, and Social Work. Perth: SAPTI WA.

Galanti G (1991) Caring for Patients from Different Cultures: Case studies from American hospitals. Philadelphia: University of Pennsylvania Press.

Gardner MF (1983) Receptive One-Word Picture Vocabulary Test. Novato CA: Academic Therapy.

Gardner MF (1990) Expressive One-Word Picture Vocabulary Test-Revised. Novato CA: Academic Therapy.

Gentile A, Ozolins U, Vasilakakos M (1996) Liaison Interpreting: A handbook. Melbourne: Melbourne University Press.

Goodman NR (1994) Intercultural education at the university level: teacher-student interaction. In RW Brislin, T Yoshida (eds) Improving Intercultural Interactions: Modules for cross-cultural training programs. Thousand Oaks: Sage Publications, pp. 129-47.

Grasska MA, McFarland T (1982) Overcoming the language barrier: problems and solutions. American Journal of Nursing, September 1376-9.

Grosjean F (1989) Neurolinguists, beware! The bilingual is not two monolinguals in one person. Brain and Language 36: 3-15.

Grosjean F (1992) Another view of bilingualism. In RJ Harris (ed.) Cognitive Processing in Bilinguals. New York: Elsevier Science Publishers, pp. 51-62.

Gudykunst WB (1993) Toward a theory of effective interpersonal and intergroup communication: an anxiety/uncertainty management (AUM) perspective. In RL Wiseman, J Koester (eds) Intercultural Communication Competence. London: Sage Publications, pp. 33-71.

Haffner L (1992) Cross-cultural medicine: a decade later. The Western Journal of Medicine 157: 255-9.

Hamers JF, Blanc MHA (1989) Bilinguality and Bilingualism. Cambridge: Cambridge University Press.

Hamilton J (1996) Multicultural health care requires adjustments by doctors and patients. Canadian Medical Association Journal 155: 585--7.

Hand L (1991) Bilingualism: everything you ever wanted to know but were afraid to ask (well . . . almost everything) — issues for speech pathologists. Australian Communication Quarterly (summer): 8-12.

Hatton DC (1992) Information transmission in bilingual, bicultural contexts. Journal of Community Health Nursing 9: 53-9.

Hatton DC, Webb T (1993) Information transmission in bilingual, bicultural contexts: a field study of community health nurses and interpreters. Journal of Community Health Nursing 10: 137-47.

Hodson BW (1984) Assessment of Phonological Processes — Spanish. San Diego: Los Amigos Research Associates.

Hornberger J, Itakura H, Wilson SR (1997) Bridging language and cultural barriers between physicians and patients. Public Health Reports 112: 410-17.

Irwin H (1996) Communicating with Asia: Understanding people and customs. St Leonards: Allen & Unwin.

Isaac K (2001a) What about linguistic diversity? A different look at multicultural health care. Communication Disorders Quarterly 22(2): 110-13.

Isaac K (2001b) Working Hand-in-Hand: Services for Culturally and Linguistically Diverse Populations. Workshop presented at Speech Pathology Australia National Conference, Melbourne, Australia.

Isaac K (2001c) Building Partnerships with Interpreters: A Research Update. Paper presented at Speech Pathology Australia National Conference, Melbourne, Australia.

Isaac K, Hand L (1996) Interpreter-mediated interactions in speech pathology: Problems and solutions. Australian Communication Quarterly (summer): 32-6.

James P (1974) James Language Dominance Test. Hingham MA: Teaching Resources.

Kanitsaki O (1993) Acute health care and Australia's ethnic people. Contemporary Nurse 2: 122-7.

Kaufert JM, Putsch RW (1997) Communication through interpreters in healthcare: ethical dilemmas arising from differences in class, culture, language, and power. The Journal of Clinical Ethics 8: 71-87.

Launer J (1978) Taking medical histories through interpreters: practice in a Nigerian outpatient department. British Medical Journal 2: 934-5.

Lee A (1989) A socio-cultural framework for the assessment of Chinese children with special needs. Topics in Language Disorders 9: 38-44.

Lidz CS, Pena ED (1996) Dynamic Assessment: The model, its relevance as a nonbiased approach, and its application to Latino American preschool children. Language, Speech, and Hearing Services in Schools 27: 367-72.

Lynch EW (1998) Developing cross-cultural competence. In EW Lynch, MJ Hanson (eds) Developing Cross-cultural Competence: A guide for working with young children and their families 2nd Ed. Baltimore: Paul H Brookes, pp. 47-89.

Lynch EW, Hanson MJ (1998) Developing Cross-cultural Competence: A guide for working with young children and their families 2nd Ed. Baltimore: Paul H Brookes.

MacLachlan M (1997) Culture and Health. Chichester: John Wiley & Sons.

Mares S (1980) Pruebas de Expresión Oral y Percepción de la Lengua Española. Downey CA: Office of the Los Angeles County Superintendent of Schools.

Mason MA, Smith BF, Henshaw MM (1976) La 'Meda': Medida Española de articulación. San Ysidro CA: San Ysidro School District.

Matsuda M (1989) Working with Asian parents: some communication strategies. Topics in Language Disorders 9: 45-53.

Mattes LJ (1987) Spanish Articulation Measures. Oceanside CA: Academic Communication Associates.

Mattes LJ (1989) Spanish Language Assessment Procedures: A communication skills inventory. Oceanside CA: Academic Communication Associates.

Mattes LJ, Omark DR (1991) Speech and Language Assessment for the Bilingual Handicapped (2 edn). Oceanside CA: Academic Communication Associates.

Meisel JM (1994) Code-switching in young bilingual children: the acquisition of grammatical constraints. Studies in Second Language Acquisition 16(4): 413-39.

Meyers C (1992) Hmong children and their families: consideration of cultural influences in assessment. The American Journal of Occupational Therapy 46: 737-44.

Miller N, Abudarham S (1984) Management of communication problems. In N Miller (ed.) Bilingualism and Language Disability: Assessment and remediation. London: Croom-Helm, pp. 192-3.

Moncada LR, Marshall MH (1982) Examenes para Diagnosticar Impedimentos de Afasia. Murfreesboro TN: Pinnacle Press.

NAATI (1999) National Accreditation Authority for Translators and Interpreters. At http://www.naati.com.au.

O'Sullivan K (1994) Understanding Ways: Communicating Between Cultures. Sydney: Hale & Iremonger.

Paradis M (1987) The Assessment of Bilingual Aphasia. Hillsdale NJ: Lawrence Erlbaum.

Patrick K (1991) Assessment of Aboriginal children: taking case histories. Australian Communication Quarterly (summer): 12-14.

Patston K (1991) Assessing bilingual aphasia: a cultural perspective. Australian Communication Quarterly (summer): 20-1.

Pauwels A (1995) Cross-cultural Communication in the Health Sciences: Communicating with migrant patients. South Melbourne: Macmillan Education Australia.

Poss JE, Rangel R (1995) Working effectively with interpreteres in the primary health care setting. Nurse Practitioner 20: 43-7.

Putsch RW (1985) Cross-cultural communication: the special case of interpreters in health care. Journal of the American Medical Association 254: 3344-8.

Roseberry CA, Connell PJ (1991) The use of an invented language rule in the differentiation of normal and language-impaired Spanish-speaking children. Journal of Speech and Hearing Research 34: 596-603.

Ruiz I (1996) Recommendations for working with interpreters. Work 6: 41-6.

Scott CJ (1997) Enhancing patient outcomes through an understanding of intercultural medicine: guidelines for the practitioner. Maryland Medical Journal 46: 175-80.

Shuy RW (1976) The medical interview: problems in communication. Primary Care 3: 365-86.

Singelis T (1994) Nonverbal communication in intercultural interactions. In RW Brislin, T Yoshida (eds) Improving Intercultural Interactions: Modules for cross-cultural training programs. London: Sage Publications, pp. 268-94.

So L (1992) Cantonese Segmental Phonology Test (research version). Hong Kong: University Department of Speech and Hearing Sciences.

Sperber D and Wilson D (1995) Relevance: Communication and Cognition (2 edn). Oxford: Blackwell Publishers.

Spitzberg BH (1991) An examination of trait measures of interpersonal competence. Communication Reports 4: 23-9.

Stevens KA, Fletcher RF (1989) Communicating with Asian patients. British Medical Journal 299: 905-6.

Thomas J (1983) Cross-cultural pragmatic failure. Applied Linguistics 4: 91-112.

Toronto AS (1973) Screening Test of Spanish Grammar. Evanston IL: Northwestern University Press.

Toronto AS (1977) Southwest Spanish Articulation Test. Austin TX: National Education Laboratory Publishers.

Toronto AS, Leverman D, Hanna C, Rosenzweig P, Maldonado A (1975) Del Rio Language Screening Test. Austin TX: National Education Laboratory.

Trudeau G (1985) Multicultural Vocabulary Test. San Diego: Los Amigos Research Associates.

Vasquez C, Javier RA (1991) The problem with interpreters: communication with Spanish-speaking patients. Hospital and Community Psychiatry 42: 163-5.

Wells S (1995) Creating a culturally competent workforce. Caring Magazine 14: 50-3.

West C (1984) Medical misfires: mishearings, misgivings, and misunderstandings in physician-patient dialogues. Discourse Processes 7: 107-34.

Woloshin S, Bickell NA, Schwartz LM, Gany F, Welch G (1995) Language barriers in medicine in the United States. Journal of the American Medical Association 273: 724-7.

Yavas M, Goldstein B (1998) Phonological assessment and treatment of bilingual speakers. American Journal of Speech-Language Pathology 7(2): 49-60.

Yavas M, Hernandorena C, Lamprecht R (1991) Avaliaçào Fonologica da Criança (Phonological Assessment of Child Speech). Porto Alegre, Brazil: Artes Medicas.

Index